D1458275

REDESIGNING CONTINUING EDUCATION IN THE HEALTH PROFESSIONS

Committee on Planning a Continuing Health Care
Professional Education Institute

Board on Health Care Services

INSTITUTE OF MEDICINE
OF THE NATIONAL ACADEMIES

THE NATIONAL ACADEMIES PRESS
Washington, D.C.
www.nap.edu

THE NATIONAL ACADEMIES PRESS   500 Fifth Street, N.W.   Washington, DC 20001

NOTICE: The project that is the subject of this report was approved by the Governing Board of the National Research Council, whose members are drawn from the councils of the National Academy of Sciences, the National Academy of Engineering, and the Institute of Medicine. The members of the committee responsible for the report were chosen for their special competences and with regard for appropriate balance.

This study was supported by Contract No. B08-03 between the National Academy of Sciences and the Josiah Macy, Jr. Foundation. Any opinions, findings, conclusions, or recommendations expressed in this publication are those of the author(s) and do not necessarily reflect the view of the organizations or agencies that provided support for this project.

International Standard Book Number-13:   978-0-309-14078-2
International Standard Book Number-10:   0-309-14078-1

Additional copies of this report are available from the National Academies Press, 500 Fifth Street, N.W., Lockbox 285, Washington, DC 20055; (800) 624-6242 or (202) 334-3313 (in the Washington metropolitan area); Internet, http://www.nap.edu.

For more information about the Institute of Medicine, visit the IOM home page at: www.iom.edu.

Printed in the United States of America

The serpent has been a symbol of long life, healing, and knowledge among almost all cultures and religions since the beginning of recorded history. The serpent adopted as a logotype by the Institute of Medicine is a relief carving from ancient Greece, now held by the Staatliche Museen in Berlin.

Suggested citation: IOM (Institute of Medicine). 2010. *Redesigning Continuing Education in the Health Professions*. Washington, DC: The National Academies Press.

"Knowing is not enough; we must apply.
Willing is not enough; we must do."
—Goethe

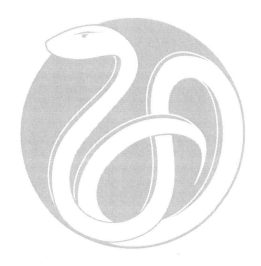

INSTITUTE OF MEDICINE
OF THE NATIONAL ACADEMIES

Advising the Nation. Improving Health.

THE NATIONAL ACADEMIES
Advisers to the Nation on Science, Engineering, and Medicine

The **National Academy of Sciences** is a private, nonprofit, self-perpetuating society of distinguished scholars engaged in scientific and engineering research, dedicated to the furtherance of science and technology and to their use for the general welfare. Upon the authority of the charter granted to it by the Congress in 1863, the Academy has a mandate that requires it to advise the federal government on scientific and technical matters. Dr. Ralph J. Cicerone is president of the National Academy of Sciences.

The **National Academy of Engineering** was established in 1964, under the charter of the National Academy of Sciences, as a parallel organization of outstanding engineers. It is autonomous in its administration and in the selection of its members, sharing with the National Academy of Sciences the responsibility for advising the federal government. The National Academy of Engineering also sponsors engineering programs aimed at meeting national needs, encourages education and research, and recognizes the superior achievements of engineers. Dr. Charles M. Vest is president of the National Academy of Engineering.

The **Institute of Medicine** was established in 1970 by the National Academy of Sciences to secure the services of eminent members of appropriate professions in the examination of policy matters pertaining to the health of the public. The Institute acts under the responsibility given to the National Academy of Sciences by its congressional charter to be an adviser to the federal government and, upon its own initiative, to identify issues of medical care, research, and education. Dr. Harvey V. Fineberg is president of the Institute of Medicine.

The **National Research Council** was organized by the National Academy of Sciences in 1916 to associate the broad community of science and technology with the Academy's purposes of furthering knowledge and advising the federal government. Functioning in accordance with general policies determined by the Academy, the Council has become the principal operating agency of both the National Academy of Sciences and the National Academy of Engineering in providing services to the government, the public, and the scientific and engineering communities. The Council is administered jointly by both Academies and the Institute of Medicine. Dr. Ralph J. Cicerone and Dr. Charles M. Vest are chair and vice chair, respectively, of the National Research Council.

www.national-academies.org

COMMITTEE ON PLANNING A CONTINUING HEALTH CARE PROFESSIONAL EDUCATION INSTITUTE

GAIL L. WARDEN (*Chair*), President Emeritus, Henry Ford Health System and Professor of Health Management and Policy at the University of Michigan, School of Public Health, Detroit

JAKO S. BURGERS, Harkness Fellow 2008-2009, Harvard School of Public Health, Boston, Massachusetts, and Senior Researcher, Scientific Institute for Quality of Healthcare (IQ healthcare), Radboud University Nijmegen Medical Centre, The Netherlands

LINDA BURNES BOLTON, Vice President and Chief Nursing Officer, Cedars-Sinai Medical Center, Los Angeles, California

CATHERINE DeANGELIS, Editor-in-Chief and Senior Vice President, Scientific Publications and Multimedia Applications, *JAMA*, Chicago, Illinois, and Professor, Johns Hopkins University, School of Medicine, Baltimore, Maryland

ROBERT D. FOX, Professor Emeritus of Adult and Higher Education, University of Oklahoma, Norman

SHERRY A. GLIED, Professor and Chair, Department of Health Policy and Management, Columbia University, Mailman School of Public Health, New York

KENDALL HO, Director, eHealth Strategy Office, Associate Professor, Division of Emergency Medicine, Faculty of Medicine, University of British Columbia, Vancouver

EDWARD F. LAWLOR, Dean and William E. Gordon Distinguished Professor, George Warren Brown School of Social Work at Washington University in St. Louis, Missouri

DAVID C. LEACH, Former Executive Director, Accreditation Council for Graduate Medical Education, Asheville, North Carolina

LUCINDA MAINE, Executive Vice President and Chief Executive Officer (CEO), American Association of Colleges of Pharmacy, Alexandria, Virginia

PAUL E. MAZMANIAN, Associate Dean for Continuing Professional Development and Evaluation Studies, School of Medicine, Virginia Commonwealth University, Richmond

MICHAEL W. PAINTER, Senior Program Officer, Robert Wood Johnson Foundation, Princeton, New Jersey

WENDY RHEAULT, Vice President, Academic Affairs, and Dean, College of Health Professions, Rosalind Franklin University of Medicine and Science, North Chicago, Illinois

MARIE E. SINIORIS, President and CEO, National Center for Healthcare Leadership, Chicago, Illinois

---

[1] Served through May 2009.

Reviewers

This report has been reviewed in draft form by individuals chosen for their diverse perspectives and technical expertise, in accordance with procedures approved by the National Research Council's Report Review Committee. The purpose of this independent review is to provide candid and critical comments that will assist the institution in making its published report as sound as possible and to ensure that the report meets institutional standards for objectivity, evidence, and responsiveness to the study charge. The review comments and draft manuscript remain confidential to protect the integrity of the deliberative process. We wish to thank the following individuals for their review of this report:

ROBERT B. BARON, University of California, San Francisco
PAUL B. BATALDEN, Dartmouth Institute for Health Policy
    and Clinical Practice
RON CERVERO, University of Georgia
COLLEEN CONWAY-WELCH, Vanderbilt University School
    of Nursing
THEODORE GANIATS, University of California, San Diego
LYNN GERBER, George Mason University
RICHARD KRUGMAN, University of Colorado, Denver
THOMAS J. MONAHAN, West Sand Lake, NY

DONALD E. MOORE, JR., Vanderbilt University School of
  Medicine
MARLA E. SALMON, University of Washington School of
  Nursing
MIKE SAXTON, Pfizer, Inc.
DAVID N. SUNDWALL, Utah Department of Health
DAVID SWANKIN, Citizen Advocacy Center
JAMES N. THOMPSON, (former) Federation of State Medical
  Boards

Although the reviewers listed above have provided many con-
structive comments and suggestions, they were not asked to endorse
the conclusions or recommendations nor did they see the final draft
of the report before its release. The review of this report was over-
seen by **NANCY ADLER,** University of California, San Francisco,
and **SUSANNE STOIBER,** Stoiber Health Policy, LLC. Appointed
by the National Research Council and Institute of Medicine, they
were responsible for making certain that an independent examination of this report was carried out in accordance with institutional
procedures and that all review comments were carefully considered.
Responsibility for the final content of this report rests entirely with
the authoring committee and the institution.

Preface

Continuing education (CE) is the process by which health professionals keep up to date with the latest knowledge and advances in health care. However, the CE "system," as it is structured today, is so deeply flawed that it cannot properly support the development of health professionals. CE has become structured around health professional participation instead of performance improvement. This has left health professionals unprepared to perform at the highest levels consistently, putting into question whether the public is receiving care of the highest possibly quality and safety.

Redesigning Continuing Education in the Health Professions is the result of the work by the Institute of Medicine (IOM) Committee on Planning a Continuing Health Care Professional Education Institute. This report does not recommend specific details about the operations of an institute—instead it illustrates a vision for a better system through a comprehensive approach of continuing professional development and a framework upon which to develop a new, more effective system. The report also offers principles to guide the creation of an institute. Refocusing the lens from CE to a system of continuing professional development supports health professionals in achieving the goal of high quality, safe health care.

CE is one of many strategies to strengthen and retool the health care workforce and just one of many pieces necessary to improve health care quality and patient safety. Yet it is a critical piece—one that has been overlooked for too long. In the current era of health reform, transformation of CE offers an actionable agenda to begin the alignment of learning with public expectations and the needs of health professionals.

I would like to extend my gratitude to the members of the committee for their commitment and dedication in developing a report based on the evidence and sound reasoning. I would also like to thank the many individuals and organizations who contributed their time to provide input to the committee's deliberations. Finally, I would like to express my appreciation to the IOM, in particular IOM senior staff and Samantha Chao, study director, for their tireless efforts.

Gail L. Warden
Chair
Committee on Planning a Continuing
Health Care Professional Education Institute
December 2009

Acknowledgments

Many individuals and organizations contributed to this study. Most specifically, the committee and staff would like to thank those experts who testified at the public workshop held on December 11, 2008, and February 12, 2009, in Washington, DC:

Cathryn Clary, Pfizer, Inc.
Linda Coogle, North American Association of Medical
    Education and Communication Companies
Jeanne Floyd, American Nurses Credentialing Center
David Gibson, Association of Schools of Allied Health
    Professions
Dwight Hymans, Association of Social Work Boards
John T. James, Patient Safety Advocate
Murray Kopelow, Accreditation Council for Continuing
    Medical Education
Patricia Lane, National Black Nurses Association and Inova
    Fairfax Hospital
Michael A. Moore, Danville Regional Medical Center
Lisa Robin, Federation of State Medical Boards
Mike Saxton, Pfizer, Inc.
Rebecca Snead, National Alliance of State Pharmacy Associations
David Swankin, Citizen Advocacy Center
Peter Vlasses, Accreditation Council for Pharmacy Education

We would also like to acknowledge the individuals who provided insight and expertise, supporting the committee's efforts throughout the report process:

Karen Adams, National Quality Forum
Neese Boston, American Psychological Association
Ashley Byrd, American Psychological Association
Stephanie J. L. Chambers, National Association of Social
    Workers Credentialing Center
Richard Cole, Federation of Chiropractic Licensing
Todd Dorman, Johns Hopkins University
Bill Dubbs, American Association for Respiratory Care
Martin Eccles, Cochrane Effective Practice and Organisation of
    Care Group
Thomas W. Elwood, Association of Schools of Allied Health
    Professions
Kelly Evans, American Therapeutic Recreation Association
Michelle Fiander, Cochrane Effective Practice and Organisation
    of Care Group
Jan Frustaglia, Association of Occupational Health
    Professionals in Healthcare
Marc Goldstein, American Physical Therapy Association
MaryAnn Gruden, Association of Occupational Health
    Professionals in Healthcare
Karen M. Hart, American Dental Association
Sarah D. Hertfelder, American Occupational Therapy
    Association
Norman Kahn, Council of Medical Specialty Societies
Gabrielle Kane, University of Washington
Alain D. Mayhew, Cochrane Effective Practice and
    Organisation of Care Group
Kathleen McGovern, Cochrane Effective Practice and
    Organisation of Care Group
Mindi McKenna, American Association of Family Physicians
Sherry Merkur, London School of Economics and Political
    Science
Greg J. Neimeyer, American Psychological Association
Karen L. Niles, American Speech-Language-Hearing
    Association
Elizabeth J. Paulsen, Cochrane Effective Practice and
    Organisation of Care Group
Laure Perrier, University of Toronto
Joan Polancic, American Society for Clinical Laboratory Science

Kate Regnier, Accreditation Council for Continuing Medical
    Education
Lisa Robin, Federation of State Medical Boards
Robert Rogers, Institute for Health Policy, Harvard Medical
    School
Corina Schmidt, American Society of Radiologic Technologists
Marcia Segura, American Psychological Association
Greg Thomas, American Academy of Physician Assistants
Dimitra V. Travlos, Accreditation Council for Pharmacy
    Education
Emma L. Wong, Nuclear Regulatory Commission

We extend special thanks to David Blumenthal and Eric Campbell, Institute for Health Policy, Harvard Medical School, and Dave Davis, Association of American Medical Colleges, who were unpaid consultants to the committee in their capacities as grantees of the Josiah Macy, Jr. Foundation. Drs. Blumenthal and Campbell offered support and advice about the financing of continuing education, most specifically about estimating the costs of continuing medical education; Dr. Davis provided guidance on lifelong learning.

Many within the Institute of Medicine were helpful to the study staff. The staff would like to thank Susan McCutchen, William McLeod, Janice Mehler, Joi Washington, and Benjamin Wheatley for their time and support to further the committee's efforts.

Finally, the committee would like to thank and recognize the support from George Thibault of the Josiah Macy, Jr. Foundation for sponsoring the study.

Contents

APPENDIXES

Boxes, Figures, and Tables

Summary

A workforce of knowledgeable health professionals is critical to the discovery and application of health care practices to prevent disease and promote well-being. Today in the United States, the professional health workforce is not consistently prepared to provide high quality health care and assure patient safety, even as the nation spends more per capita on health care than any other country. The absence of a comprehensive and well-integrated system of continuing education (CE) in the health professions is an important contributing factor to knowledge and performance deficiencies at the individual and system levels.

To be most effective, health professionals at every stage of their careers must continue learning about advances in research and treatment in their fields (and related fields) in order to obtain and maintain up-to-date knowledge and skills in caring for their patients. Many health professionals regularly undertake a variety of efforts to stay up to date, but on a larger scale, the nation's approach to CE for health professionals fails to support the professions in their efforts to achieve and maintain proficiency.

In one attempt to better understand the possibilities for improving CE, the Josiah Macy, Jr. Foundation convened a conference in 2007 that brought together stakeholders in health care and continuing health professional education. Agreeing that the current state of CE in the United States is inadequate, the stakeholders recommended that a national interprofessional continuing education institute be created and charged with "advancing the science

BOX S-1
Statement of Task

An ad hoc IOM committee will undertake a review of issues in continuing education (CE) of health care professionals that are identified from the literature and from data-gathering meetings with involved parties to improve the quality of care. Based on this review, the committee will consider the establishment of a national interprofessional CE Institute to advance the science of CE by promoting the discovery and dissemination of more effective methods of educating health professionals over their professional lifetimes, by developing a research enterprise that encourages increased scientific study of CE, by developing mechanisms to assess research applications, by stimulating new approaches to both intra- and interprofessional CE, by being independent and composed of individuals from the various health professions, and by considering financing (both short and long term).

of CE." In response, the foundation asked the Institute of Medicine (IOM) to review issues related to the continuing education of health professionals and to consider the establishment of a national interprofessional institute dedicated to improving CE (see Box S-1). The IOM appointed the Committee on Planning a Continuing Health Care Professional Education Institute. In this report, the committee examines CE for all health professionals,[1] explores development of a national continuing education institute, and offers guidance on the establishment and operation of such an institute. In order to add perspective to its deliberations, the committee examined a number of possible alternatives to an institute, and the report describes some of the pros and cons of the various options. The report provides five broad messages:

- **There are major flaws in the way CE is conducted, financed, regulated, and evaluated.** As a result, the health care workforce is not optimally prepared to provide the highest quality of care to patients or to meet public expectations for quality and safety.
- **The science underpinning CE for health professionals is fragmented and underdeveloped.** These shortcomings have

---

[1] Health professionals were identified here as those health care practitioners and technical occupations classified by the Bureau of Labor Statistics that require baccalaureate or higher degrees for licensure.

made it difficult if not impossible to identify effective educational methods and to integrate those methods into coordinated, broad-based programs that meet the needs of the diverse range of health professionals.

- **Continuing education efforts should bring health professionals from various disciplines together in carefully tailored learning environments.** As team-based health care delivery becomes increasingly important, such interprofessional efforts will enable participants to learn both individually and as collaborative members of a team, with a common goal of improving patient outcomes.
- **A new, comprehensive vision of professional development is needed to replace the culture that now envelops continuing education in health care.** Such a vision will be key in guiding efforts to address flaws in current CE efforts and to ensure that all health professionals engage effectively in a process of lifelong learning aimed squarely at improving patient care and population health.
- **Establishing a national interprofessional CE institute is a promising way to foster improvements in CE for health professionals.** This report proposes the creation of a public-private entity that involves the full spectrum of stakeholders in health care delivery and continuing education and that is charged with developing and overseeing comprehensive change in the way CE is conducted, financed, regulated, and evaluated.

THE CURRENT STATE OF CONTINUING EDUCATION

For health professionals, continuing education encompasses the period of learning from postlicensure to career's end. CE is intended to enable health professionals to keep their knowledge and skills up to date, with the ultimate goal of helping health professionals provide the best possible care, improve patient outcomes, and protect patient safety.

The reality of continuing education, however, is far different. Although there are instances of programs focused on those goals, on an overarching level the U.S. approach to CE has many flaws:

- Health professionals and their employers tend to focus on meeting regulatory requirements rather than identifying personal knowledge gaps and finding programs to address them. Many of the regulatory organizations that oversee CE tend not to look beyond setting and enforcing minimal, narrowly defined competencies.

- The current approach to CE is most often characterized by didactic learning methods, such as lectures and seminars; traditional settings, such as auditoriums and classrooms; specific (frequently mandated) intervals; and teacher-driven content that may or may not be relevant to the clinical setting.
- CE is operated separately in each profession or specialty, with responsibility dispersed among multiple stakeholders within each of those communities.
- The scientific literature offers guidance about general principles for CE but provides little specific information about how to best support learning; for the most part, CE providers cannot determine the effectiveness of their instructional methods, and health professionals lack a dependable basis for choosing among CE programs. Further, the inability to draw definitive conclusions about the effectiveness of specific CE methods has clouded discussions about the larger value of continuing education for health professionals.
- In medicine and pharmacy—and nursing to some extent— pharmaceutical and medical device companies have taken a lead role in financing the provision of and research on CE. Such commercial funding has raised and continues to raise concerns about conflicts of interest and whether some companies are using CE to influence health professionals so as to increase market share.
- Regulations vary widely by specialty and by state, as state boards generally are responsible for determining the number of CE credits required for profession-specific *licensure*. *Certification* and *credentialing*, two other major parts of the regulatory environment, are characterized by wide variations as well. *Accreditation* of CE providers may be based on an evaluation of the quality of specific CE activities or of CE providers. Such wide variations in CE regulation lead to inconsistent learning and conflict with efforts to achieve high levels of competence and practice for every health professional.

TOWARD A SYSTEM OF CONTINUING
PROFESSIONAL DEVELOPMENT

The hallmarks of a well-prepared health professional have been delineated in several previous IOM reports. *Crossing the Quality*

Chasm: A New Health System for the 21st Century calls on health professionals to provide care that is safe, effective, patient-centered, efficient, timely, and equitable. *Health Professions Education: A Bridge to Quality* recommends that all clinicians possess five core competencies, which include being able to provide patient-centered care, work in interprofessional teams, employ evidence-based practice, apply quality improvement, and utilize informatics. Together, these quality goals represent the foundation for building a better continuing education system.

Requirements that are based on credit hours rather than outcomes—and that vary by state and profession—are not conducive to teaching and maintaining these core competencies aimed at providing quality care. Improving the system for CE will therefore require changes that expand its conventional boundaries.

An emerging concept, called continuing professional development (CPD), includes components of CE but has a broader focus, such as teaching how to identify problems and apply solutions, and allowing health professionals to tailor the learning process, setting, and curriculum to their needs. The principles of CPD already have been adopted in numerous other countries, including the United Kingdom and other members of the European Union, Canada, and New Zealand. Some groups in the United States, including the American Medical Association and the Accreditation Council for Pharmacy Education, also have recognized the broader learning opportunities that CPD offers and have adopted the concept as a guide. In line with such examples, the committee adopted the term CPD to signal the importance of multifaceted, lifelong learning in the lives of all health professionals.

In this new vision, a CPD system takes a holistic view of health professionals' learning, with opportunities stretching from the classroom to the point of care. It shifts control of learning to individual health practitioners and has the flexibility to adapt to the needs of individual clinicians, enabling them to be the architects of their own learning. The system bases its education methods on research theory and findings from a variety of fields, and embraces information technologies to provide professionals with greater opportunities to learn effectively.

If coordinated nationally and across the health professions, a CPD system offers the promise of advancing evidence-based, interprofessional, team-based learning; engendering coordination and collaboration among the professions; providing higher quality for a given amount of resources; and leading to improvements in patient health and safety.

A NATIONAL CONTINUING PROFESSIONAL
DEVELOPMENT SYSTEM

The committee ultimately concluded that a continuing professional development institute offered the most promise for redress-
ing the flaws in the current approach to CE. But first the committee
considered five potential routes for creating an effective system
for CPD.

1. *Status quo.* While some beneficial learning is taking place
   under the status quo, the flaws documented in this report cannot be remedied by anything short of a coordinated national
   effort.
2. *New program within an existing government agency.* The committee considered placing responsibility for a national CPD
   system in either the Agency for Healthcare Research and
   Quality or the Health Resources and Services Administration,
   which both fund health care research. Placing responsibility
   for a national CPD system in one of these agencies would tie
   CPD to either improved quality or more team-based care.
   However, a federal program could not as readily incorporate
   collaborative decision-making, including public and private
   sector actors, and could also be subject to procedural and/or
   financial requirements that could diminish its effectiveness.
3. *Ad hoc coalition of current stakeholders and organizations.* A broad
   coalition of stakeholders could create a national interprofessional CPD system. The committee specifically considered
   a coalition that includes current stakeholders and organizations whose purposes are to improve health care quality and
   patient safety (e.g., National Committee for Quality Assurance and the National Quality Forum). Expanding to the req-
   uisite breadth will require a strong central convener; reducing
   professional and state variability is beyond the ability of such
   an ad hoc group for the foreseeable future.
4. *A private structure operated by professional societies and organizations.* Such a structure could include all health professions
   and develop collaborations with other stakeholders (e.g.,
   employers, researchers, state boards, funders) to build the
   remaining infrastructure needed to support a CPD system.
   Two features missing from this approach are an incentive to
   convene and an oversight body for accountability.
5. *A new public-private structure.* Like the purely private structure, a public-private organization could catalyze participation of a broad set of stakeholders in improving health care

quality and patient safety, but it would also be accountable to the federal government. Of the five alternatives, creating a new organization with so many interested parties will be complicated.

The committee concluded that alternative 5, establishing a public-private body that would promote collaboration among a variety of stakeholders and be held accountable by the federal government, offers the most promise. By fostering collaboration among diverse groups, it could develop and oversee a comprehensive research agenda that would reach across health professions; it could serve to coordinate current licensure, certification, credentialing, and accreditation activities and encourage the groups in charge to work toward regulatory standards for CPD that reflect research findings. Collectively, the stakeholders could develop and adopt broad conflict-of-interest policies and identify new and more consistent funding sources for CPD to replace conflicted funding.

The committee therefore calls on the federal government to work with stakeholders and act as the initial convener of efforts to develop a public-private institute devoted to improving continuing professional development that will foster the delivery of high quality health care.

Recommendation 1: The Secretary of the Department of Health and Human Services should, as soon as practical, commission a planning committee to develop a public-private institute for continuing health professional development. The resulting institute should coordinate and guide efforts to align approaches in the areas of:
(a) Content and knowledge of CPD among health professions,
(b) Regulation across states and national CPD providers,
(c) Financing of CPD for the purpose of improving professional performance and patient outcomes, and
(d) Development and strengthening of a scientific basis for the practice of CPD.

The remainder of this report refers to the proposed public-private institute as the Continuing Professional Development Institute (CPDI). An effective CPD system would offer significant improvement over today's fragmented approach to continuing education. In designing an institute that will accomplish the broad goals of Recommendation 1, the planning committee will need to consider how to achieve each of the components of an effective CPD system.

Recommendation 2: To achieve the new vision of a continuing professional development system, the planning committee should design an institute that:

(a) Creates a new scientific foundation for CPD to enhance health professionals' ability to provide better care;

(b) Develops, collects, analyzes, and disseminates metrics, including process and outcome measures unique to CPD;

(c) Encourages development and use of health information technology and emerging electronic health databases as a means to provide feedback on professionals' and health system performance;

(d) Encourages development and sharing of improvement tools (e.g., learning portfolios and assessment resources) and theories of knowledge and practice (e.g., peer review systems for live documentation, such as wikis) across professions;

(e) Fosters interprofessional collaboration to create and evaluate CPD programs and processes; and

(f) Improves the value and cost-effectiveness of CPD delivery and considers ways to relate the outputs of CPD to the quality and safety of the health care system.

A central tenet of this report is that collaboration among various stakeholders, including patients and members of the public, is essential to developing an improved CPD system. By working together, the CPD community and the health care quality improvement community will be best able to drive more efficient resource allocation and increase the overall value of CPD.

Recommendation 3: The planning committee should design the Continuing Professional Development Institute to work with other entities whose purpose is to improve quality and patient safety by:

(a) Collaborating with the Agency for Healthcare Research and Quality, the Centers for Medicare and Medicaid Services, the Joint Commission, the National Committee for Quality Assurance, the National Quality Forum, and other data measurement, collection, cataloguing, and reporting agencies to evaluate changes in the performance of health professionals and the need for CPD in the improvement of patient care and safety; and

(b) Involving patients and consumers in CPD by using patient-reported measures and encouraging transparency to the public about performance of health care professionals.

Advancing the Science of CPD

The current body of literature does not conclusively identify the most effective CE methods, the correct mixture of CE methods, or the amount of CE needed to maintain competence or to improve clinical outcomes. The literature does offer some guidance for improved learning, suggesting that CE should be guided by needs assessments, should be interactive, and should provide multiple learning opportunities and multiple methods of education.

Future research needs to include identifying theoretical frameworks, determining proven and innovative CPD methods and the degrees to which they apply in various contexts, defining CPD outcome measures, and determining influences on learning. The fields of adult learning, education, sociology, psychology, organizational change, systems engineering, and knowledge translation can support the advancement of how CPD should be provided.

Recommendation 4: The Continuing Professional Development Institute should lead efforts to improve the underlying scientific foundation of CPD to enhance the knowledge and performance of health professionals and patient outcomes by:
 (a) Integrating appropriate methods and findings from existing research in a variety of disciplines and professions,
 (b) Generating research directions that advance understanding and application of new CPD solutions to problems associated with patient and population health status,
 (c) Transforming new knowledge pertinent to CPD into tools and methods for increasing the success of efforts to improve patient health, and
 (d) Promoting the development of an inventory of measurement instruments that can be used to evaluate the effectiveness and efficiency of CPD.

Collecting and Disseminating Data

The data required to assess a health professional's educational needs, identify effective programs to meet those needs, and evaluate CPD programs are derived from a diverse range of professional fields and geographic locations. As a result of gaps in data collection, validation, and analysis, decisions about continuing education and professional development are often not based on evidence. Specifically, data should help determine what effectively influences a health professional's capacity to deliver high quality health care.

Recommendation 5: The Continuing Professional Development Institute should enhance the collection of data that enable evaluation and assessment of CPD at the individual, team, organizational, system, and national levels. Efforts should include:

(a) **Relating quality improvement data to CPD, and**
(b) **Collaborating with the Office of the National Coordinator for Health Information Technology in developing national standardized learning portfolios to increase understanding of the linkages between educational interventions, skill acquisition, and improvement of patient care.**

Enhancing the Effectiveness of Regulation

The effectiveness of CPD programs is influenced by every aspect of regulation—i.e., the licensure, certification, and credentialing of health professionals and the accreditation of CPD providers. At present, the fragmentation and variation that now characterize the regulatory landscape inhibit development of a system that systematically improves professionals' competence and performance across the entire continuum of CPD.

Current regulators have the knowledge and expertise to assess learning and continuing education activities. However, their efforts are "siloed" and ineffective in achieving consistently high quality CE. The role of a national interprofessional organization is to promote collaboration across the entire CPD regulatory system, with the ultimate goal of improving health care quality and patient safety. The CPDI should work with current regulatory bodies to establish national standards that can underpin stronger systems.

Recommendation 6: The Continuing Professional Development Institute should work with stakeholders to develop national standards for regulation of CPD. The CPDI should set standards for regulatory bodies across the health professions for licensure, certification, credentialing, and accreditation.

Improving Financing

Adequate and assured long-term financial support for the Continuing Professional Development Institute and CPD research will be necessary to realize a fully developed CPD system. Although no data exist to project whether the costs of a comprehensive CPD system would be greater or less than the costs of the current system, the committee's judgment is that sufficient funding exists within the current structure to support better learning.

Efforts to eliminate or avoid conflicts of interests in the funding of CPD, such as practitioner-sponsored CPD and the pooling of funds contributed by various parties already are under way. By building on these, the planning committee and the CPDI would be well positioned to develop and adopt national guidelines on conflicted sources of funding for all health professions.

Recommendation 7: The Continuing Professional Development Institute should analyze the sources and adequacy of funding for CPD, develop a sustainable business model free from conflicts of interest, and promote the use of CPD to improve quality and patient safety.

Health care often benefits when professionals from within and across disciplines work together. But in many situations today, care may not be practiced in teams because people are not trained in teams. Interprofessional experiments have resulted in pockets of programs whose experiences can be incorporated into better CPD. A shared educational framework can align communication and share advances across all health professions.

Recommendation 8: The Continuing Professional Development Institute should identify, recognize, and foster models of CPD that build knowledge about interprofessional team learning and collaboration.

Before they are ready for widespread adopting, new methods for providing continuing professional development must prove their effectiveness through rigorous testing (e.g., demonstration programs). A number of innovative CPD methods remain at that stage. For example, learning portfolios, which are development tools that document professionals' progress of their practice skills, can be used across professions, but their effectiveness in improving the learning process and health professional performance must be assessed. Demonstration programs can be developed using the research and development structures currently in place.

Recommendation 9: Supporting mobilization of research findings to advance health professional performance, federal agencies that support demonstration programs, such as the Agency for Healthcare Research and Quality and the Health Resources

and Services Administration, should collaborate with the Continuing Professional Development Institute.

By its very nature, continuing professional development will be complex, involving many stakeholders playing various roles. Continuous evaluations therefore will be needed to ensure that progress is being made toward better health professional development. Evaluation could occur at four levels that will require different metrics: individual health professionals, stakeholder organizations, the Continuing Professional Development Institute, and the overall CPD system. Arguably, the most important but most difficult level of evaluation is that of the overall CPD system. To hold the CPDI accountable for its activities and stewardship of the CPD system, the institute should be required to make periodic reports, analogous to Medicare Payment Advisory Commission (MedPAC) reports, to the Secretary. The institute should provide its first report after 2 to 5 years of operation, to allow for the usual problems that typically occur in any new venture.

> **Recommendation 10: The Continuing Professional Development Institute should report annually to its public and private stakeholders and should hold a national symposium on the performance and progress of professional development and its role in enhancing quality of care and patient safety.**

GUIDELINES FOR PLANNING AND STRUCTURING THE CONTINUING PROFESSIONAL DEVELOPMENT INSTITUTE

The Planning Committee

In implementing the recommendations in this report, the planning committee will need to define the Continuing Professional Development Institute's scope of work, develop a governance model, identify sources of financing, and identify and manage relationships with current and new stakeholders—including determining the extent of the federal role in the public-private institute. The committee should operate under four basic principles. It should be held accountable by the public and the Secretary. It should be competency-based, flexible, and nimble. It should broadly communicate with and gather input from the rest of the field (e.g., professional societies, accreditors, CPD providers, licensing bodies), but make decisions based only on the votes of the committee members. Finally, it should use consensus building, not parliamentary procedure, in developing processes.

The committee should be funded by contracts and grants from the government and private foundations to support staff and travel. The IOM committee envisions the planning committee to consist of 13-15 members. The members should be recognized leaders in their respective fields, have experience in leading change and improvement, and have some level of experience in interprofessional learning. At a minimum, membership should include practicing professionals and individuals with expertise in CPD research and government. The committee should be led by a chair who has a record of success in setting and implementing visions and building consensus.

The Institute

The CPDI should be an independent body with membership and financing from both the public and the private sectors. The federal government initially should oversee and coordinate the development of the CPDI, and a competency-based board should be appointed to lead the CPDI's activities. Ultimately, upon the decision of the institute's board, the government's responsibilities should be transferred back to CPD stakeholders. Unless the board determines otherwise, the Secretary will eventually have no formal role in the institute. The size of the CPDI's budget should depend on its exact functions and breadth, and its budget should be initially projected by the planning committee and refined by the board.

The planning committee should determine the structure of the CPDI's initial board, its membership size, and the competencies that need to be represented among board members. Several members of the planning committee should be named to the board, in order to facilitate the institute's transition from planning to implementation. Once the board has achieved a more permanent structure, its members should rotate off in an overlapping manner.

Considering the breadth of issues addressed by the CPDI, the board may find it valuable to establish a number of standing councils and ad hoc committees as needed. The committee suggests four initial standing councils on issues identified in this report—on the science of CPD, on regulation, on financing, and on data collection and dissemination. The councils would involve a larger group of diverse stakeholders in raising issues and providing advice to the board, and would add transparency to the CPDI's planning and operations.

CONCLUSION

Developing and implementing a new national system to improve continuing professional development on a broad scale, across disciplines and government boundaries, will be difficult but offers the best hope for addressing the host of problems that prevent CE from adequately serving health professionals, patients, and the nation. To help catalyze the transition to a better CPD system—one that is coordinated, harmonized, and efficient—the federal government can play a key role as a central convener, bringing together diverse stakeholders in health care and continuing education who collectively can shape a new national interprofessional institute. In turn, the institute, in collaboration with stakeholders, will be centrally positioned to foster a new CPD system that can prepare all health professionals to perform to their highest potential. Working together, these forces can fulfill the vision of ensuring that the nation has a workforce of health professionals who can provide high quality, safe care and improve patient outcomes.

1

Continuing Professional Development: Building and Sustaining a Quality Workforce

The health care system in the United States falls short of its goal of consistently providing the best possible care. The nation spends more on health care than any other country in the world—and too often receives care of mediocre quality that is too frequently unsafe. Actions taking place at the local, state, and national levels—most recently through the development of the White House Office of Health Care Reform—show some promise for providing greater access to safe, high quality care for all Americans. Such actions include promotion of systems improvement, measurement and reporting activities of health care processes and outcomes, public engagement, and realignment of payment systems. But these efforts typically overlook a critical piece of improving quality: developing and maintaining a reliable, properly trained health professional workforce. A well-educated workforce is critical to the discovery and application of health care practices to prevent disease, promote well-being, and increase the quality life-years of the public.

THE ROLE OF HEALTH PROFESSIONALS IN IMPROVING QUALITY

Health professionals serve as the bridge between patients, the knowledge generated by scientific research, and the policies and practices to implement that knowledge. As the recipients of care,

15

the public trusts health professionals to provide care that is safe, efficient, effective, timely, patient-centered, and equitable.

The health professions covered by this report are those listed by the Bureau of Labor Statistics as "healthcare practitioner and technical occupations" with baccalaureate or higher degrees (see Appendix B). Examples of included professions are physicians, physician assistants, dentists, dieticians, nurses, and speech-language pathologists. These health professionals undergo extensive formal education, followed by what has become known in the United States as continuing education (CE). CE lasts the duration of a health professional's career and is therefore the model of learning that spans the longest period. It serves two functions: maintenance of current practice and translation of knowledge into practice.

Educating professionals about new theories and evidence of what does and does not work, and under what circumstances, is one part of promoting the provision of better health care. Because individual learning styles differ greatly, innovative learning methods are developed to help health professionals maintain their competencies. Over time, learning methods have evolved from a focus on professionals' attendance at and satisfaction with a limited set of educational activities to a focus on demonstrably changing professional practice and improving patient outcomes. Better learning methods need to be developed continuously, as creating appropriate methods, processes, and contexts is imperative for professionals to provide the highest quality care possible. Health professionals also need to provide feedback to themselves and the system about what actually works in specific practice settings, as the common wisdom of what "should be" practiced continuously evolves. What is considered to be the best knowledge one day may later be found to be inadequate. Health professionals' abilities to identify these instances and adapt is critical. With the development of the Internet and Web 2.0, the world of information has expanded at exponential rates—so much so that the breadth of information for which health professionals used to be responsible is now beyond the capacity of any one professional.

On average, it now takes 14-17 years for new evidence to be broadly implemented (Balas and Boren, 2000). Shortening this period is key to advancing the provision of evidence-based care, and will require the existence of a well-trained health professional workforce that continually updates its knowledge.

TRAINING, EDUCATION, AND
PROFESSIONAL DEVELOPMENT

Lifelong learning is the notion that learning occurs along a continuum, from elementary and secondary education to undergraduate and graduate education, lasting through the end of one's career. There are several stages of learning, including training, education, and professional development. These terms are used somewhat interchangeably, but clear distinctions should be made due to their varying abilities to both promote and confine learning. Training often refers to the standardization of a process to yield similar results. Education refers to the process by which people learn to apply solutions to problems and adapt to new situations. Professional development transcends both concepts and includes areas such as self-directed learning, systems changes, and quality improvement; it teaches people not only how to apply solutions but also how to focus on actual performance and how to identify problems.

Within this schematic, continuing education is largely teacher-driven, focuses on clinical education, and predominantly builds on education theory. CE often is associated with didactic learning methods, such as lectures and seminars, which take place in auditoriums and classrooms. In theory, the purpose of continuing education is to update and reinforce knowledge, which should ultimately result in better patient care. But in practice, there often are conflicting ideas about the purpose of CE. Some health professionals see CE as a means to attain credits for the licensure and credentialing they need to practice their occupations. Employers often view CE as a way to keep staff up to date and to improve quality. Many regulators believe the purpose of CE is to maintain competence and improve quality.

In recent years, a broader concept, called continuing professional development (CPD), has been emerging that incorporates CE as one modality while adding other important features. CPD is learner-driven, allowing learning to be tailored to individual needs. CPD uses a broader variety of learning methods and builds on a broader set of theories than CE. CPD methods include self-directed learning and organizational and systems factors; and it focuses on both clinical content and other practice-related content, such as communications and business. Although CPD is a relatively new term to some U.S. health professionals, the term is used widely in Canada, New Zealand, and the European Union, including the United Kingdom (see Appendix C). CPD encompasses more diverse learning formats than those in CE (e.g., clinical reminders and academic detailing, where practitioners learn about drug prescribing from noncommercial sources) (Davis et al., 2003), and takes place in more diverse settings, such as clinical settings. CPD can be defined as the system for maintaining, improving, and broadening knowledge and skill throughout one's professional life. CPD is focused squarely on promoting effective practice, and is better positioned than other stages of learning to effect change because it occurs when professionals are most likely to be aware of their needs. It also integrates content and educational design for individual practitioners in the practice setting.

Given its narrower focus, CE can limit a health professional's learning, as it does not seem to offer the broader opportunities for learning that CPD does. As some groups have already done (e.g., Accreditation Council for Pharmacy Education, American Medical Association), this report adopts the term CPD to recognize the importance of more comprehensive, lifelong learning. In the context of this report, CPD is used to address the future state and CE is used when addressing past and current continuing education efforts, even though some elements of CPD are being used in limited contexts. Table 1-1 illustrates the various features of training, education, and professional development, including continuing professional development.

TABLE 1-1 Comparing Training, Education, and Professional Development

	Training	Education	Professional Development
Purpose	"To impart a set of established facts and skills without the necessity of [a] trainee's understanding why [he] should act in the prescribed manner" (Carney, 2003)	"To introduce, review, or alter knowledge and competencies" (Fox, 2003)	To encourage systematic maintenance, self-directed improvement, and broadening of knowledge and skills
Targets	A uniform, predictable behavior	Altered knowledge, skill, or attitudes	Outcomes-focused development of personal and professional qualities necessary through a professional career or life

TABLE 1-1 Continued

	Training	Education	Professional Development
Outcomes	Passive activity; conditioned reflex action	Observation, analysis, and questioning to formulate hypotheses and make conclusions; actions modified according to conclusions or solutions	Reflecting on practice, identifying problems
		Continuing Education	Continuing Professional Development (CPD)
Description		Serves to update and reinforce knowledge (e.g., management of heart attacks, diagnosis of HIV)	Deals with personal, communication, managerial, and team-building skills in addition to content
		Frequently based on acquiring credits	May be based on acquiring credits or on processes of self-accreditation and reflection (e.g., personal portfolios)
		May be considered a subset of continuing professional development	Systems for monitoring CPD require flexibility so professionals can participate in a variety of CPD activities

HISTORICAL CONTEXT

Continuing education has long been a core part of being a health professional, beginning with Florence Nightingale encouraging nurses to continue to learn (Gallagher, 2006) and the first recorded continuing nursing education course dating back to 1894 (Stein, 1998). In medicine, CE was often confused with graduate medical education in the 1920s and 1930s as a way to address the issue of improperly trained physicians, but this ended with the advent of internship and residency, which extended formal physician training. After World War I, medical faculties became increasingly concerned with the need to spur professional growth of physicians in practice, and continuing medical education (CME) was used as a way to help well-trained practitioners keep up to date with the advancing knowledge. Although reports from the 1930s and 1940s called for the continuation of medical education beyond undergraduate and graduate level education, it was not until after World War II that these calls were acted on (Commission on Graduate Medical Education, 1940; Shepherd, 1960). Today's construct of using CME to improve performance began in the late 1970s when CME was suggested to be a continuous process based in practice settings (Lloyd and Abrahamson, 1979).

Calls for the professionalization of medicine have also significantly impacted medical education. One of the first studies about physicians' preferred continuing education methods crystallized the need to better identify effective CE methods and courses (Vollan, 1955). The objectives and competencies needed to be learned by medical students and other health professionals that shape today's health professions education were not clearly delineated until recently (AAMC, 1998; IOM, 2003).

In addition to the changing context and goals of CE, its structure has also evolved. In medicine, changes to residency programs required greater faculty attention, and there arose a growing sense among faculty that teaching CME was less than prestigious. In the 1950s, studies showed that pharmaceutical sales representatives were the most important sources providing physicians with new information; this trend led to the development of a new industry tying together pharmaceutical companies, advertising, and physician behavior. This new industry soon became subject to criticism about the potential conflicts of interest between pharmaceutical companies and physicians, and such issues have been the focus of periodic congressional hearings since the 1960s (Randall, 1991; United States Senate Committee on Finance, 2007; United States Senate Subcommittee on Antitrust and Monopoly, 1962). Regulation of

CME began largely as a method for the American Medical Association, and eventually state medical societies, to monitor pharmaceutical influence on physician education. As a result, CME increasingly came to be provided by a combination of specialty societies, state and local medical organizations, and pharmaceutical companies (Ludmerer, 1999; Podolsky and Greene, 2008). Health professionals are currently regulated by state health licensing boards; providers of CE are regulated by national accrediting organizations (e.g., National League of Nursing).

The CE industry has grown rapidly over the past 10 years and has increasingly involved commercial support from the medical education and communication companies that began appearing in the early 1980s. Continuing medical education activities have become increasingly extravagant (Podolsky and Greene, 2008), raising questions not only of the effectiveness of the education being provided but also of the level of influence commercial entities should have on physician learning. Currently, financial support, accreditation mechanisms, and CE methods are intertwined and difficult to analyze separately in medicine. Limited data also suggest that similar trends are taking place in nursing and pharmacy but not in the allied health professions.

Significant change in health professions education is not unprecedented. Specific to medicine, the report *Medical Education in the United States and Canada*, better known as the Flexner Report, was published in 1910. The report dramatically changed the culture and landscape of medical education and became the basis of undergraduate medical education in the United States. At the time of the Flexner report, many observers were concerned that there were too many medical schools and that physicians were being poorly trained. There also were concerns about the perceived lack of standardized prerequisites and curriculums across medical schools; the reliance on education through lectures and memorization, not at a patient's bedside; and the proprietary nature of medical education. These concerns about undergraduate medical education in the early 1900s mirror today's concerns about the continuing education of all health professions, as highlighted in the report *Work and Integrity* (Campbell and Rosenthal, 2009; Cooke et al., 2006; Flexner, 1910; Sullivan, 2005).

STUDY CONTEXT

Continuing education differs widely among and within health professions in terms of content, delivery or learning methods, regulation, and financing. Currently, CE is largely driven by state requirements and regulatory bodies that often focus on number of hours spent in CE courses, calculated in terms of some units for all professions. But even this basic measure differs markedly across states. For example, physicians in Alabama are required to have 12 CME credits per year, while those in Michigan need 50 credits per year, and many states have no requirement at all. Some states require a minimum number of credits in ethics, while others require mandatory content such as courses in infectious disease and patient safety. Depending on the state, annual hours or credit requirements differ among professions: nurses generally need 5-15 contact hours, pharmacists need 10-60 hours, and when required, social workers need anywhere between 3 and 25 hours. A greater problem, however, compounds the variations in CME requirements among states and professions: current data is insufficient to determine how much CE is really needed to maintain competence, to support learning, or to affect performance. This gap brings into question the current regulatory focus on credits and hours.

How learning is best achieved is another question to be addressed when evaluating CE. Potential sources for better learning methods may lie in the field of adult education research and theory. Research in such areas as andragogy, experiential learning, self-directed learning, lifelong learning, and critical reflection may offer information that can be incorporated in designing CE delivery methods. Methods for delivering CE vary widely and include more traditional methods such as conferences, grand rounds, and published materials. As technology has improved, the various types of computer-based and Internet-based learning modes have evolved to include interaction with CD-ROMs, webinars, and videoconferences. CE is now also delivered within the context of care, often termed practice-based learning and point-of-care learning. Maximizing learning is critical to developing a better system of continuing professional development.

Regulation of how much and what type of CE health professionals must obtain is conducted at the federal, state, and local levels through licensure and certification, which set the minimum standards of competency for a profession. In most cases, professionals must receive a license before they are allowed to practice. Licensure and relicensure requirements vary by profession and generally vary by state. Certification is provided by professional societies and boards, which acknowledge competence in a particular specialty, often requiring more in-depth knowledge than licensure. Credentialing occurs at the level of the health care organization and verifies that a health professional has received training up to the level required by the organization. Accreditation is provided by organizations often associated with professional organizations that evaluate programs delivering CE to individual health professionals.

A major problem that stems from this fragmented system is that many of the regulatory agencies do not work together, although there is a recent trend toward collaboration among some professions. The regulatory system ought to consider placing emphasis on the relationship between quantity of hours or CE activities, practitioner performance, and clinical outcomes, both for individual professionals and for organizations.

The CE industry is funded in part by professionals, professional societies, professional schools, publishing/education companies, and the health care delivery system. Medicine is the largest of the professions in terms of CE income, with more than $2.5 billion of total income in 2007. Commercial funds represent more than 50 percent of total CME income, or $1.5 billion. Physician membership organizations, publishing/education companies, and schools of medicine have the largest profit margins of all CME organizations, with profit margins of 46.6 percent, 34.9 percent, and 13.8 percent, respectively (ACCME, 2008). In social work and allied health, continuing education is often paid for by professionals themselves and not reimbursed by employers, although data are scarce about the many allied health professions.

A critical assessment of the effectiveness of CE on the performance of health professionals is needed at the individual and aggregate discipline levels, on the various modes of CE delivery, and on the ability of health professionals to close the gap between current and optimal health system performance. This assessment is made difficult, however, by the relative lack of high quality studies in the published literature. Importantly, no evidence exists to determine exactly how much CE is needed for professionals to, at a minimum, maintain competence and practice at the highest level.

STUDY CHARGE AND APPROACH

In 2007, the Josiah Macy, Jr. Foundation held a conference to discuss the future of continuing health professions education (Hager et al., 2007). The conference, which brought together a diverse set of stakeholders, concluded that CE in the United States is currently inadequate. The conference summary states that CE currently is more focused on numbers of credits than on health professionals' actual performance, is funded in large part by organizations with conflicted interests, is not focused on learning based in practice and patient care, does not provide incentives for interprofessional care, and does not take advantage of advances in Internet technology. Conference attendees recommended that a continuing education institute be created for the purpose of "advancing the science of CE" and that the Institute of Medicine (IOM) appoint a committee to discuss the development of such an institute. The Macy Foundation subsequently asked the IOM to review issues in continuing education and consider the establishment of a national interprofessional continuing education institute (see Box 1-1). In response, the IOM convened the Committee on Planning for a Continuing Health Professional Education Institute.

In accordance with its statement of task, the IOM study committee reviewed a variety of issues surrounding the state of continuing education for health professionals, but did not try to identify specific educational methods or approaches to be used in CE. The committee focused only on postlicensure learning, although it recognizes the importance of strengthening the entire continuum of health professional learning. Using its review findings as a basis, the committee considered issues that would relate to the establishment of a national CE institute, including how such an institute might best be established and how it should operate. Despite the inclusion of "Institute" in its name, the committee examined a number of possible alternatives to establishing an institute and considered whether the objectives of the institute could be met with a different organizational structure.

BOX 1-1
Statement of Task

An ad hoc IOM committee will undertake a review of issues in continuing education (CE) of health care professionals that are identified from the literature and from data-gathering meetings with involved parties to improve the quality of care. Based on this review, the committee will consider the establishment of a national interprofessional CE Institute to advance the science of CE by promoting the discovery and dissemination of more effective methods of educating health professionals over their professional lifetimes, by developing a research enterprise that encourages increased scientific study of CE, by developing mechanisms to assess research applications, by stimulating new approaches to both intra- and interprofessional CE, by being independent and composed of individuals from the various health professions, and by considering financing (both short and long term).

The Macy Foundation approved two other grant proposals at the same time it approved the IOM study. The first of these grants was awarded to the Association of American Medical Colleges (AAMC), in collaboration with the American Association of Colleges of Nursing, to hold a stakeholders workshop to discuss the translation of CE research findings into practice. The workshop, held in February 2009, resulted in a paper made publicly available in fall 2009 (AAMC and AACN, 2010). The second grant was awarded to the Institute for Health Policy at Harvard University to conduct economic modeling for alternative financing models for continuing medical education, and the researchers presented their findings in a white paper (Campbell and Rosenthal, 2009). The IOM committee considered in its deliberations the information presented in both papers, but the committee developed its conclusions and recommendations independently and reported its findings to the Macy foundation separately.

IOM Committee Methods

The committee met three times during the course of the 12-month study and conducted a literature review on the effectiveness of continuing education methods (see Appendix A). The committee also received public statements from a large variety of stakeholders, including regulatory bodies, funders, health professionals, and consumers. Representatives from medicine, pharmacy, nursing, social work, and allied health professions provided statements to the committee at a public workshop (see Appendix E), sharing their perspectives on the purpose of CE and the need for change. These statements and others received during the committee's process were instrumental to the development of this report.

Previous IOM Reports

This report builds on and is consistent with previous IOM reports that have emerged from a 10-year quest to identify ways to improve the quality of care that patients receive, improve patient outcomes, and better protect patient safety. The call to improve quality and patient safety was sounded by *To Err Is Human: Building a Safer Health System* (1999) and expanded by *Crossing the Quality Chasm: A New Health System for the 21st Century* (2001a). As a central theme, these reports cited the need to improve the quality of the health professional workforce. Other IOM studies dealing with the health care workforce have focused on specific care settings (e.g., long-term care [IOM, 2001b]), specific populations (e.g., aging [IOM, 2008], children and family [IOM, 2000]), and specific disciplines (e.g., mental health and substance use [IOM, 2006], rural health [IOM, 2005], and public health [IOM, 2007d]). A number of studies on nursing and emergency care professionals also concluded that their workforces must be strengthened (IOM, 2004, 2007a, 2007b, 2007c).

The current report also draws in important ways on the IOM report *Health Professions Education: A Bridge to Quality* (2003), which identified five core competencies that all health professionals should have and made recommendations for improving the testing and assurance of health professionals' competencies. The five core competencies include being able to provide patient-centered care, work in interdisciplinary teams, employ evidence-based practice, apply quality improvement strategies, and use health informatics.

REPORT STRUCTURE

Across its breadth, this report illustrates the importance of changing the current CE system and provides principles that will help in moving to a broad-based continuing professional development system over the next 10 years.

The report is organized into seven chapters, of which this introductory chapter is the first. Chapter 2 discusses the scientific foundations of continuing education and includes a critical assessment of the effectiveness of CE methods. Chapter 3 explores CE regulation and financing. Chapter 4 builds a case for improving continuing education and explores the various alternatives to a CE institute. Chapter 5 discusses what a better CE system would look like in 10 years. Chapter 6 describes the function and structure of a continuing professional development institute, and Chapter 7 explores steps toward the implementation, research, and evaluation of such an institute. Recommendations and conclusions are embedded within each chapter.

REFERENCES

AAMC (Association of American Medical Colleges). 1998. *Learning objectives for medical student education: Guidelines for medical schools.* https://services.aamc.org/publications/showfile.cfm?file=version87.pdf&prd_id=198&prv_id=239&pdf_id=87 (accessed September 4, 2009).
AAMC and AACN (American Association of Colleges of Nursing). 2010. *Lifelong learning in medicine and nursing: Final conference report.* http://www.aamc.org/meded/cme/lifelong/macyreport.pdf (accessed January 13, 2010).

ACCME (Accreditation Council for Continuing Medical Education). 2008. *AC-CME annual report data 2007*. http://www.accme.org/dir_docs/doc_upload/207fa8e2-bdbe-47f8-9b65-52477f9faade_uploaddocument.pdf (accessed January 16, 2009).

Balas, E., and S. Boren. 2000. Managing clinical knowledge for health care improvement. *Yearbook of Medical Informatics*. Stuttgart: Schattaver Verlagsgesellschaft.

Campbell, E. G., and M. Rosenthal. 2009. Reform of continuing medical education: Investments in physician human capital. *Journal of the American Medical Association* 302(16):1807-1808.

Carney, A. L. 2003. Factors in instructional design: Training versus education. Presented at the Instructional Technology Lab Seminar at the University of Illinois, Chicago.

Commission on Graduate Medical Education. 1940. *Graduate medical education*. Chicago: University of Chicago Press.

Cooke, M., D. M. Irby, W. Sullivan, K. M. Ludmerer. 2006. American medical education 100 years after the Flexner Report. *New England Journal of Medicine* 355(13):1339-1344.

Davis, D., M. Evans, A. Jadad, L. Perrier, D. Rath, D. Ryan, G. Sibbald, S. Straus, S. Rappolt, M. Wowk, and M. Zwarenstein. 2003. The case for knowledge translation: Shortening the journey from evidence to effect. *British Medical Journal* 327(7405):33-35.

Flexner, A. 1910. *Medical education in the United States and Canada*. New York: Carnegie Foundation for the Advancement of Teaching.

Fox, R. D., ed. 2003. *Encyclopedia of education, second edition*. Edited by J. W. Guthrie. New York: Macmillan Reference USA.

Gallagher, L. 2006. Continuing education in nursing: A concept analysis. *Nurse Education Today* 27(8).

Hager, M., S. Russell, and S. Fletcher. 2007. *Continuing education in the health professions: Improving healthcare through lifelong learning*. Proceedings of a conference sponsored by the Josiah Macy, Jr. Foundation, Bermuda, November 28-December 1. New York: Josiah Macy, Jr. Foundation.

IOM (Institute of Medicine). 1999. *To err is human: Building a safer health system*. Washington, DC: National Academy Press.

———. 2000. *From neurons to neighborhoods: The science of early childhood development*. Washington, DC: National Academy Press.

———. 2001a. *Crossing the quality chasm: A new health system for the 21st century*. Washington, DC: National Academy Press.

———. 2001b. *Improving the quality of long-term care*. Washington, DC: National Academy Press.

———. 2003. *Health professions education: A bridge to quality*. Washington, DC: The National Academies Press.

———. 2004. *Keeping patients safe: Transforming the work environment of nurses*. Washington, DC: The National Academies Press.

———. 2005. *Quality through collaboration: The future of rural health*. Washington, DC: The National Academies Press.

———. 2006. *Improving the quality of health care for mental and substance-use conditions*. Washington, DC: The National Academies Press.

———. 2007a. *Emergency medical services at the crossroads*. Washington, DC: The National Academies Press.

———. 2007b. *Emergency medical services for children: Growing pains*. Washington, DC: The National Academies Press.

———. 2007c. *Hospital-based emergency care: At the breaking point*. Washington, DC: The National Academies Press.

———. 2007d. *Training physicians for public health careers*. Washington, DC: The National Academies Press.

———. 2008. *Retooling for an aging America: Building the health care workforce*. Washington, DC: The National Academies Press.

Lloyd, J. S., and S. Abrahamson. 1979. Effectiveness of continuing medical education: A review of the evidence. *Evaluation Health Professions* 2:20.

Ludmerer, K. 1999. *Time to heal*. New York: Oxford University Press.

Podolsky, S. H., and J. A. Greene. 2008. A historical perspective of pharmaceutical promotion and physician education. *Journal of the American Medical Association* 300(7):831-833.

Randall, T. 1991. Kennedy hearings say no more free lunch—or much else—from drug firms. *Journal of the American Medical Association* 265(4):440-442.

Shepherd, G. R. 1960. History of continuation medical education. *Journal of Medical Education* 35(8):740-758.

Stein, A. M. 1998. History of continuing nursing education in the United States. *Journal of Continuing Education in Nursing* 29(6):245-252.

Sullivan, W. M. 2005. *Work and integrity: The crisis and promise of professionalism in America (2nd edition)*. The Carnegie Foundation for the Advancement of Teaching. San Francisco: Josey-Bass.

United States Senate Committee on Finance. 2007. *Committee staff report to the chairman and ranking member: Use of educational grants by pharmaceutical manufacturers*. Washington, DC: U.S. Government Printing Office.

United States Senate Subcommittee on Antitrust and Monopoly. 1962. *Report on administered prices: Drugs*. Washington, DC: U.S. Government Printing Office.

Vollan, D. D. 1955. Scope and extent of postgraduate medical education in the United States. *Journal of the American Medical Association* 157(9):703-708.

2

Scientific Foundations of Continuing Education

In 1967, the National Advisory Committee on Health Manpower recommended that professional associations and government regulatory agencies take steps to ensure the maintenance of competence in health professionals (U.S. Department of Health, Education, and Welfare, 1967). To support this objective, states in the 1970s began to mandate that health professionals receive continuing education (CE). Requirements were applied unevenly across the United States, however, and there now is variability from state to state and profession to profession regarding how much CE is needed, what kind of CE is needed, and how and when CE should be administered (Landers et al., 2005). In the late 1970s, many observers argued that the time was ripe for change in the CE system, and they raised a number of important questions: Can CE guarantee competence? Are mechanisms available to accurately assess the learning needs of health professionals? How can these learning needs best be met? How many annual contact hours are needed to ensure competence? (Mazmanian et al., 1979). Today, it is clear that this call for change went unanswered. CE has evolved organically, without an adequate system in place to ensure that the fundamental questions raised three decades ago could be addressed to inform the development and maintenance of a CE system. These still-relevant questions provide a springboard toward creating a more responsive and comprehensive system.

Pressure from a number of groups, including the Pew Taskforce on Health Care Workforce Regulation (1995) and the Institute of Medicine (IOM), has spurred debate about how best to ensure the continuing competence of health professionals. As discussed in Chapter 1, the IOM report *Health Professions Education: A Bridge to Quality* (2003) details five core competencies deemed necessary for all health professionals: patient-centered care, interdisciplinary team-based care, evidence-based practice, quality improvement strategies, and the use of health informatics. These competencies are intended to help provide a more safe, effective, patient-centered, efficient, timely, and equitable health care system (IOM, 2001). For example, advances in the areas of evidence-based practice and quality improvement require the ability to integrate clinical knowledge with professional practice. Connecting these processes through evidence-based health professional education has the potential to revolutionize the health care system (Berwick, 2004; Cooke et al., 2006).

The components of CE—the CE research system, regulatory and quasi-regulatory bodies, and financing entities—are currently ill-equipped to support these core competencies consistently. For example, as this chapter later details, effective CE incorporates feedback and interaction, yet 76 percent of continuing medical education (CME) instruction hours are delivered through lectures and conferences (ACCME, 2008) that typically limit interactive exchange (Forsetlund et al., 2009). Various professions, however, have begun to use different methods of CE, including methods that better take into account the clinical practice setting (Kues et al., 2009; MacIntosh-Murray et al., 2006).

Research on CE methods and theories behind adult learning, education, sociology, psychology, organizational change, systems engineering, and knowledge translation have provided an initial evidence base for how CE and continuing professional development *should* be provided. Additionally, previous works have offered theoretical frameworks for conceptualizing CE and guiding its provision (Davis and Fox, 1994; Fox et al., 1989).

This chapter presents summary data on the ways in which CE is typically provided. The chapter discusses the most common methods of providing CE; details findings on the effectiveness of CE in general, as well as the effectiveness of specific CE methods; discusses theories that support what is known about how adults learn; and describes the attributes of successful CE methods and how theory can be applied to improve these methods.

METHODS OF PROVIDING CONTINUING EDUCATION

In its current form, CE consists primarily of didactic activities that are not always related to clinical settings or patient outcomes. Lectures and conference sessions, long the mainstay of CE, remain the most commonly used CE methods (see Figure 2-1). For physicians, courses and regularly scheduled series (e.g., grand rounds) account for 44.1 percent of total reported activities conducted by providers accredited by the Accreditation Council for Continuing Medical Education (ACCME) and 88.1 percent of total activities presented by providers accredited by state medical societies (ACCME, 2008). More than 82 percent of total hours of instruction are in the form of courses or series.

The committee made a concerted effort to incorporate data regarding methods of CE delivery from all health professions; however, the data collected for most professions are not robust and are not always reported in comparable formats. Consequently, publicly available data on pharmacy, nursing, dentistry, physical therapy, and other allied health professions' CE are much more limited than in medicine.

In 2007-2008, the Accreditation Council for Pharmacy Education (ACPE) accredited 36,569 activities. Of these, 53 percent were "live activities," 46 percent were home study, and 11 percent were Internet activities.[1] The category of live activities includes lectures, symposia, teleconferences, workshops, and webcasts, but the percentage of each of these activities is unknown. For licensed social workers, survey participation rates provide some insight into the types of CE most often used (Table 2-1). Social workers, like physicians and pharmacists, often participate in formal, didactic workshops. Informal CE activities such as peer consultation, which may not be counted for CE credit by state licensing boards, are the methods most believed by social workers to change their practice behavior (Smith et al., 2006). In many health professions, journal reading is a commonly used avenue to complete CE credits.

CE providers are increasingly using an expanding variety of CE methods. A 2008 survey of academic CME providers found an "increasing diversity" of offerings beyond traditional, didactic conferences, courses, and lectures (Kues et al., 2009, p. 21). CE programs more often use multiple educational methodologies (e.g., interaction, experiential learning) and multiple educational techniques (e.g., questioning, discussion, coaching, role play). Table 2-2 provides a

---

[1] Personal communication, D. Travlos, ACPE, June 2, 2009.

32

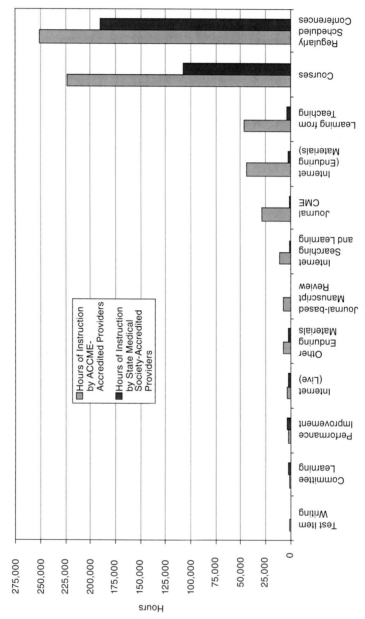

FIGURE 2-1 Accredited methods of CE by hours of instruction.
SOURCE: ACCME, 2008.

TABLE 2-1 Methods of CE Reported by Social Workers

Activity	Participation Rates	
	%	N
Workshops	97.0	223
Peer consultation	76.5	176
Reading books or journals	73.5	169
In-service training	66.1	152
Supervision or mentoring	47.4	109
Academic courses	7.8	18

SOURCE: Smith et al., 2006.

list of common approaches. Data on the use of these approaches are not always available. For example, the rate at which health professionals participate in self-directed learning is not available from CE providers or accreditors because in most health professions, CE credits—the metric for CE activities—cannot currently be earned for participation in self-directed learning.

The use of e-learning has become increasingly widespread in the training of health professionals. e-Learning modalities include educational programs delivered via electronic asynchronous or real-time communication without the constraints of place, or, in some cases, time (Wakefield et al., 2008). Although some professionals prefer traditional learning formats that include more face-to-face contact (Jianfei et al., 2008; Sargeant et al., 2006), e-learning has the advantage of enabling health professionals to set their own learning pace, review content when needed, and personalize learning experiences (Harden, 2005). Lower costs, potentially greater numbers of participants, and increased interprofessional collaborations are additional benefits of e-learning (Bryant et al., 2005). e-Learning can facilitate, for example, interprofessional team-based simulation training (Segrave and Holt, 2003). The ways in which various formats of e-learning may be used in professional practice are summarized in Table 2-3.

DEFINING OUTCOME MEASURES

Assessing the effectiveness of CE methods requires clarifying desired outcomes. Traditionally, efforts to measure CE effectiveness were constrained by a lack of consensus around ideal measures for evaluating CE learning outcomes (Dixon, 1978). Participation rates, satisfaction of participants, and knowledge gains—as evaluated by postactivity exams—were used to show that participants in a CE

TABLE 2-2 Common Approaches to Providing CE

Method	Description
Experiential and self-directed learning	A professional's experience factors into learning activities; the structure, planning, implementation, and evaluation of learning are initiated by the learner (Davis and Fox, 1994; Stanton and Grant, 1999)
Reflection	An individual marks ideas, exchanges, and events for teaching-learning (Fox et al., 1989; Schön, 1987)
Academic detailing	Outreach in which health professionals are visited by another knowledgeable professional to discuss practice issues
Simulation	The act of imitating a situation or a process through something analogous. Examples include using an actor to play a patient, a computerized mannequin to imitate the behavior of a patient, a computer program to imitate a case scenario, and an animation to mimic the spread of an infectious disease in a population
Reminders	Paper or computer-generated prompts about issues of prevention, diagnosis, or management delivered at the time of care and point-of-care
Protocols and guidelines	A set of rules generated by piecing together research-based evidence in the medical literature, representing the optimal approaches to managing a medical disease
Audit/feedback	Health care performance is measured and the results are presented to the professional
Multifaceted methods	Comprehensive programs designed to improve health professional performance or health care outcomes using a variety of methods
Educational materials	Publications or mailings of written recommendations for clinical care, including guidelines and educational computer programs
Opinion leaders	Individuals recognized by their own community as clinical experts with well-developed interpersonal skills
Patient-mediated strategies	Techniques that increase the education of patients and health consumers (e.g., health promotion media campaigns, directed prompts)

TABLE 2-3 Examples of e-Learning

Computer or Internet	Simulation	EHR and EMR	Portable Computing
• Internet-based case discussions • Mixed mode (live + web) • Webinars • Clinical practice guidelines • Practice reminders • InfoPOEMS • Social networking, Web 2.0 • Knowledge co-creation • Micro- or macro-system dashboards • Data representation and reflection	• Web case simulations • Lo- or hi-fidelity simulations • Team-based simulation exercises • System modeling • Care mapping	• Self-audit of case series • Learning portfolios • Individual dashboards • Pop-up case-sensitive dialogue boxes • Interprofessional EHRs • PACS • System audits • e-portfolios	• Podcasting • 3G videos • Smart phone-based videoconferencing • Decision support tools (e.g., ePocrates, Up-to-Date) • Smart phone-based social networking tools

NOTE: 3G = 3rd generation wireless communications; EHR = electronic health record; EMR = electronic medical record; PACS = picture archival communications system.

activity had reached at least the "knows" outcome level indicated in Table 2-4. The science of measuring outcomes is advancing beyond measuring procedural knowledge as researchers have come to focus on linking CE to patient care and population health (Miller, 1990; Moore et al., 2009; Tian et al., 2007). An effective CE method is now understood to be one that has enhanced provider performance and thus improved patient outcomes (Moore, 2007).

The relationships among teaching, learning, clinician competence, clinician performance, and patient outcomes are difficult to measure (Jordan, 2000; Mazmanian et al., 2009; Miller, 1990) and complicated by the inherent challenges in measuring actual, not just potential or reported, behavior. In health care settings, it may remain difficult to measure dependent variables (Eccles et al., 2005) because linking participation in CE to changes in the practice set-

TABLE 2-4 Continuum of Outcomes for Planning and Assessing CE Activities

Miller (1990)	Moore et al. (2009)	Description
	Participation	The number of health professionals who participated in the CME activity
	Satisfaction	The degree to which the expectations of the participants about the setting and delivery of the CME activity were met
Knows	*Learning*: Declarative knowledge	The degree to which participants are able to state what the CE activity intended them to know
Knows how	*Learning*: Procedural knowledge	The degree to which participants are able to state how to do what the CE activity intended them to know how to do
Shows how	Competence	The degree to which participants show in an educational setting how to do what the CE activity intended them to be able to do
Does	Performance	The degree to which participants do in their practices what the CE activity intended them to be able to do
	Patient health	The degree to which the health status of patients improves due to changes in the practice behavior of participants
	Community health	The degree to which the health status of a community of patients changes due to changes in the practice behavior of participants

SOURCE: Adapted from Moore et al., 2009.

ting is a complex process that cannot easily be tracked using current methods. Additionally, the provision of interprofessional care makes it difficult to attribute the education of one professional to a patient outcome (Dixon, 1978). Furthermore, due to the nature of some types of professional work, such as social work, evaluating outcomes of client-professional interaction is inherently difficult if not ethically impossible (Griscti and Jacono, 2006; Jordan, 2000).

Continuing education is concerned with both health professional learning processes and broader outcomes, including patient outcomes and organizational change. Therefore, CE is itself part of a complex learning system and relies on evidence-based research that is driven by theory. Theories are developed over time and continuously build on evidence-based practice, practice-based learning, and outcomes. However, the transition between research and practice is often difficult. Closing the gaps between research and practice, as depicted in Figure 2-2, may be achieved by blending clinical practice and knowledge (MacIntosh-Murray et al., 2006).

In the absence of data on patient outcomes, health professionals' self-reported knowledge gains and behavior change resulting from participation in a CE activity may provide insight into learning. In some cases, self-reported gains have been shown to reflect actual behavior change (Curry and Purkis, 1986; Davis et al., 2006; Parker III and Mazmanian, 1992; Pereles et al., 1997; Wakefield et al., 2003), but self-reported knowledge gains and behavior change may not always be accurate and valid (Gordon, 1991). Self-reports

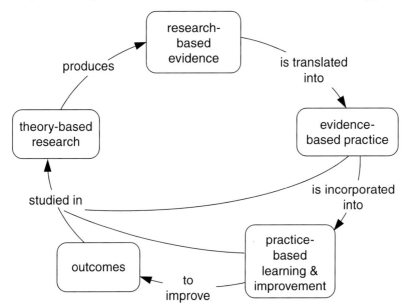

FIGURE 2-2 Closing the research-practice gaps for health care professionals and continuing education professionals.
SOURCE: MacIntosh-Murray et al., 2006.

afford health professionals a voice in evaluating themselves and their motivations. Although self-reports should never be the sole basis for decision making regarding the general effectiveness of continuing education, they may serve important purposes by enabling CE providers to identify motivations and gaps in knowledge (Eva and Regehr, 2008; Fox and Miner, 1999).

MEASURING THE EFFECTIVENESS OF CONTINUING EDUCATION

The effectiveness of continuing education has been researched, debated, and discussed for decades. An oft-cited review of CME found that the weakness of most published evaluations limited possible conclusions about the effectiveness of CME (Bertram and Brooks-Bertram, 1977), while a seminal review of eight studies provided evidence that formal CME helped physicians improve their clinical performance (Stein, 1981). Soon after publication of that review, however, a benchmark study in the *New England Journal of Medicine* stated that "CME does not work" (Sibley et al., 1982). To evaluate these contradictory statements and findings in the contemporary context, the committee reviewed evidence on the effectiveness of CE methods. The committee synthesized results from a literature search of more than 18,000 articles from fields including CE, knowledge translation, interprofessional learning and practice, and faculty development in three rounds of detailed assessment of each study's design, method, outcomes, and conclusions. A total of 62 studies and 20 systematic reviews and meta-analyses relevant to CE methods, cost-effectiveness, or educational theory were included (see Appendix A). Studies from a variety of health professions were included.

The literature review revealed that researchers have used a range of research designs to address a broadly defined research agenda, but the research methods used generally were weak and often lacked valid and reliable outcome measures. Several authors (Davis et al., 1999; Marinopoulos et al., 2007; O'Brien et al., 2001; Wensing et al., 2006) have questioned the propriety of systematic reviews as a tool for CE research due to a lack of a widely accepted taxonomy for the comparability of CE methods. Indeed, for several decades, authors have maintained that data on CE effectiveness are limited because studies of CE methods do not uniformly document the major elements of the learning process (Stein, 1981). Although 29 of the evaluated studies were randomized controlled trials assessing changes in clinical practice outcomes based on participation in a CE method, none had been validated through replication. While controlled trial methods produce quantifiable end points, they do not fully explain whether outcomes occur as a result of participation in CE (Davis et al., 1999); thus, a variety of research methods may be necessary. Cohort and case-control designs may be more appropriate (Mazmanian and Davis, 2002). In general, more robust research methods must be developed and used to assess CE effectiveness adequately.

Research studies measuring outcomes in terms of behavior, clinical behavior, and/or patient outcomes were generally weak in quality and results. Of the 62 studies reviewed, 8 used patient outcomes (e.g., mortality, smoking cessation, cardiac complications) to assess a health professional's learning resulting from participation in a CE activity. In lieu of CE outcomes measures linked directly to patient outcomes, self-reported behavior change was used to assess effectiveness in 9 of the 62 studies. Fourteen studies used the prescribing process to determine changes in prescription trends that may have resulted from a health professional's participation in a CE activity.

Overall Effectiveness of CE

Although CE research is fragmented and may focus too heavily on learning outside of clinical settings, there is evidence that CE works, in some cases, to improve clinical practice and patient outcomes. For example, a seminal, qualitative study of physicians explored how physicians change, finding that CME can be a "force for change" within a comprehensive strategy for learning (Fox et al., 1989). A recent, comprehensive analysis of CME identified 136 articles and 9 systematic reviews summarizing the evidence regarding CME effectiveness in imparting knowledge and skills, changing attitudes and practice behavior, and improving clinical outcomes (Marinopoulos et al., 2007). Although this analysis could not determine the effectiveness of all CME methods covered, CME was found, in general, to be effective for acquiring and sustaining knowledge, attitudes, and skills, for changing behaviors, and for improving clinical outcomes. Some evidence has supported the overall effectiveness of CE in specific instances (Davis et al., 1995; Fox, 2000; Mazmanian and Davis, 2002; Robertson et al., 2003), but too little evidence exists to make a compelling case for the effectiveness of CE, under specific circumstances.

Effectiveness of Specific CE Methods

The findings of several notable studies (Davis et al., 1992, 1995, 1999; Grimshaw et al., 2002; Grol, 2002; Grol and Grimshaw, 2003) are in general agreement that some methods are more "predispose[d] toward success" than others (Slotnick and Shershneva, 2002). The committee's review, like other reviews on CE effectiveness, provides only limited conclusions about the effectiveness of specific methods. Some tentative insights include:

Interactive techniques, such as academic detailing and audit/ feedback, generally seem effective. Previous research has indicated that interactive workshops can result in moderately large changes in professional practice behavior, compared with didactic presentations (O'Brien et al., 2001). Print media, such as self-study posters, were generally ineffective. Methods that included multiple exposures to activities tend to produce more positive results than one-time methods, a finding aligned with previous studies indicating that health professionals are more likely to apply what they have learned in practice if they participate in multiple learning activities on a single topic (Davis and Galbraith, 2009; Davis et al., 1992, 1995; Mansouri and Lockyer, 2007; Marinopoulos et al., 2007; Mazmanian et al., 2009).

Simulations appear to be effective in some instances but not in others. Simulations to teach diagnostic techniques generally are more effective than simulations to teach motor skills. Assessing the effectiveness of simulation is complicated by the diversity of simulation types, ranging from case discussions to high-fidelity simulators.

e-Learning offers opportunities to enhance learning and patient care; however, without a comprehensive body of evidence, judging the effectiveness of e-learning methods is difficult. The methods for evaluating e-learning effectiveness are relatively weak, which makes demonstrating the effect of e-learning on patient outcomes difficult. Data may emerge, however, as technology and metrics are further enabled (Cook et al., 2008; Fordis et al., 2005; Maio et al., 2003; Pui et al., 2005; Wutoh et al., 2004). Ultimately, e-learning may be equal to or better than more traditional learning methods for individual health professionals, as measured by learner satisfaction and their acquisition of knowledge and skills.

THEORETICAL UNDERPINNINGS OF CONTINUING EDUCATION

There is a 40-year history of conceptualizing CE (Cervero, 1988; Eraut, 2001; Houle, 1980; Nowlen, 1988). The earliest model, called the "update model," was built on methods of teaching, with a different educational model to develop evidence about the ways in which adults learn (Miller, 1967). Since then, research has focused on how adult learning is best accomplished, for example, by involving learners in identifying and solving problems. Considerations of context have also been addressed, particularly regarding how conditions shape CE in practice. One example is the concept that adult learners are influenced by a "double helix" of professional performance shaped by individual ability within complex organizational and cultural circumstances (Nowlen, 1988, p. 73). Many researchers have elaborated and extended this practice-based CE model (Cervero, 1988; Eraut, 1994, 2001; Houle, 1980; Nowlen, 1988), and practice-based learning is now at the forefront of educational agendas throughout the professions (Cervero, 2001; Moore and Pennington, 2003). The principal emphasis is no longer on content but rather on what is attained in knowledge, skills, attitude, and improved performance at the end of a learning activity.

The design of CE activities should be guided by theoretical insights into how learning occurs and what makes the application of new knowledge more likely. Insights can be drawn from the literature of several academic disciplines, including adult education, sociology, psychology, knowledge translation, organizational change, engineering, and systems learning (Bennett et al., 2000). However, CE providers too often fail to base their methods on theoretical perspectives (Olson et al., 2005), despite the fact that many of the most effective CE methods have a theoretical basis in adult education (Carney, 2000; Hartzell, 2007; Mann et al., 2007; Pinney et al., 2007; Pololi et al., 2001).

Select Theories on Learning

A range of theoretical perspectives have been offered on how adults learn (Merriam, 1987; Merriam and Caffarella, 2007). These perspectives cover such topics as what motivates a person to begin a lifelong learning process and how the relevance of the learned material impacts the amount of knowledge that will be retained. Table 2-5 describes several theories of learning that have been influential in shaping adult education.

Lifelong Learning

Experience is a valuable component of lifelong learning. CE is a dynamic process—moving from inquiry to instruction to

TABLE 2-5 Overview of Select Theories of Learning

Lifelong learning	An approach to learning whereby health professionals continually engage in learning for personal goals
Theories of motivation	A body of theories (e.g., discrepancy analysis, proficiency theory) explaining intrinsic motivations for engaging in learning
Self-directed learning	An approach to learning whereby the structure, planning, implementation, and evaluation of learning are initiated by the learner
Reflection	A learning tool in which an individual evaluates how experiences can guide action
Experiential learning	An approach to learning whereby a health professional's experiences are seen as an educational resource

performance—that continues throughout a health professional's career (Houle, 1984). Inquiry might start with a health professional's identification of a clinical question; instruction is the process through which knowledge or skills are then disseminated. Lifelong learning includes formal and informal modes of instruction, such as reflection, casual dialogue with peers, and lectures. CE outcomes may be best achieved when the instruction results in a health professional "internalizing an idea or using a practice habitually" (Houle, 1980, p. 32).

Through the process of lifelong learning, health professionals become aware of the reasoning and evidence that underlie their beliefs, biases, and habits (King and Kitchener, 1994). This approach to learning, in which health professionals continually engage in learning for their own personal goals, is in contrast to simply participating in formal CE for the purposes of receiving credit (King and Kitchener, 1994). Lifelong learners are sophisticated and complex. Therefore, theorists have sought to explain the implications of these complexities for the provision of CE to health professionals (Davis, 2004; Davis and Simmt, 2003; Davis and Sumara, 2006; Doll, 1993; Osberg, 2005). Complex learners are influenced by their own knowledge base as well as by their collaborative relationships with others.

Teachers of complex learners must therefore attend to these various components of influence (McMurtry, 2008).

Learning experiences are construed by health professionals in light of previous experiences and influences from other professionals and with regard to wider social processes. Thus, CE involves not only explicit curricular goals, but also recognition of unpredictable interactions, ideas, and relationships that emerge from professionals and CE providers. This kind of CE curriculum might, for example, favor collective learning that incorporates and builds on the variety of backgrounds, interests, knowledge, abilities, and personalities within a typical community of practice. The curriculum might favor a dynamic in which the CE provider and the health professional participate together rather than working under a more basic teacher-driven approach (Davis and Simmt, 2003).

Theories of Motivation

Health professionals themselves can influence the effectiveness of CE activities through the attitudes they take during the experience and the methods they select (Moon, 2004). Motivation may come from an external source, such as the need to satisfy CE requirements, or from an internal source, such as curiosity and a desire to learn. A number of theories, including discrepancy analysis, seek to explain the origins of this type of intrinsic motivation. In discrepancy analysis, for example, the learner is assumed to become motivated when he senses a discrepancy between things as they are and things as they ought to be. The learner seeks to increase competency through learning, thereby restoring balance and bringing what is and what ought to be closer in line (Fox and Miner, 1999).

A number of other theories, including proficiency theory, suggest that gaps in knowledge may produce discomfort and therefore motivation to change. Proficiency theory holds that motivation rises when a person sees a gap between the desired level of proficiency and his own (Knox, 1990; Merriam, 1987; Merriam and Caffarella, 2007). A clinician's ability to carry out learning and change is also related to his degree of confidence in his own abilities. The learner's sense of self-efficacy—the belief in his own ability to meet prospective challenges—impacts learning because those with greater self-efficacy are likely to make greater efforts and persist longer in seeking to learn (Bandura, 1977).

Self-directed Learning

If health professionals choose to learn only as problems arise, they may not be performing critical self-examinations to identify situations before they become problematic. Therefore, internal needs assessment, in which adult learners assess their own learning needs, plays a role in learning. The underlying theory behind self-directed learning comes from Knowles' theoretical assumptions regarding adult learners (see Table 2-6). Self-directed learning offers opportunities for health professionals to assess their previous experiences and existing knowledge and then set learning goals, locate resources, decide on which learning methods to use, and evaluate processes (Brookfield, 1995). Self-directed learners thus are more purposeful, motivated, and reactive (Knowles, 1975).

Self-directed learning activities are meant to be more closely tailored to the needs of the learner than activities that are controlled and directed by others. Individuals, because they are "inherently self-regulating," can and do identify clinical questions, set their own learning goals, develop strategies to address them, implement actions, and evaluate the success of those approaches (Mann and Ribble, 1994, p. 71). Evidence suggests that adults consistently seek to direct their own learning (Fox et al., 1989; Long, 1997) and that they plan and direct self-learning projects on a regular basis (Tough, 1971).

The central motivations that lead physicians, for example, to initiate learning include a desire for enhanced competence, the perception that their clinical environment presses for a change, and social pressures relating to relationships to colleagues in the same institution or profession. Additionally, professionalism, which is an internalized set of socially generated expectations, is a powerful agent for change (Fox et al., 1989). These findings indicate that comparing a health professional's performance against that of his peers can be a facilitator in identifying learning needs.

TABLE 2-6 Theoretical Assumptions of Andragogy: "The Art and Science of Helping Adults Learn"

1. Adults move toward self-direction as they mature (i.e., they become more independent)

2. Experience is a resource for learning

3. Motivations to learn are oriented to the usefulness of the knowledge

4. Orientation to learning shifts from subject-centered to problem-centered

SOURCE: Knowles, 1980.

Reflection

Reflection is a learning tool with implications for the teaching-learning process (Schön, 1983, 1987), particularly for health professionals who must learn from practice (Benner and Tanner, 1987). Professionals, despite operating in "zones of mastery," sometimes face unique and complex situations that are not resolved by using habitual practices (Schön, 1983). Through reflection, health professionals can incorporate new knowledge into practice.

Two different methods of reflection can facilitate learning: reflection-in-action and reflection-on-action. Through reflection-in-action, a health professional can reframe the experience to determine if or how it fits with his existing knowledge base (Schön, 1983, 1987). Reflection-in-action, which has been termed "thinking on your feet," problem solving, and "single-loop learning," involves looking to experiences, especially when workplace pressure prevents a professional from asking questions or admitting he does not know (Bierema, 2003; Smith, 2001). In contrast, reflection-on-action, also termed "double-loop learning," occurs when evaluating how an experience can guide action (Argyris, 1991; Schön, 1983). Teaching health professionals to engage in reflection-on-action is a key component in developing the skills necessary to be a self-directed learner.

The point at which a health professional does not know the answer—the point at which he can engage in reflective practice—is a teachable moment that may be ignored by health professionals who are unaware of or choose not to use reflection and self-assessment (Davis et al., 2006; Eva et al., 2004; Hill, 1976). Teachable moments, which are also referred to as clinical questions, are essential to health professionals' learning (Moore and Pennington, 2003). Learning may best occur in the context of patient care when it is directly applicable to clinical questions (Ebell and Shaughnessy, 2003).

Habits, frames of reference, feelings, and value judgments can influence the way a professional thinks, acts, and reflects (Mezirow, 1990). For example, a recurrent theme in cognitive research on decision making is that humans are prone to biases. In CE, this might indicate a change in perspective: CE providers may show the pervasive nature of biases and instruct professionals how to recognize the infrequent situations in which biases tend to fail (Regehr and Norman, 1996). Reflection allows health professionals to become aware of these underlying assumptions and biases, influencing how thinking and action occur.

Experiential Learning

The start and end of any teachable moment or period of reflection should involve self-assessment through which the professional critically reflects on how the learning experience should inform future decisions about both clinical care and learning (Gibbs, 1988). Experiential learning informs a health professional's experiences with theory about what should be done (Stanton and Grant, 1999). The cycle of experiential learning begins and ends in active experiences that include the planning, learning, and application of new knowledge (Dennison and Kirk, 1990; Kolb, 1984). The planning phase may include needs assessment and curriculum design, while the learning phase itself may incorporate a variety of educational methods, such as peer appraisal, self-reflection, case studies, and role play (Stanton and Grant, 1999). Experiential learning is based on the idea that teaching should be grounded in learners' experiences and that these experiences represent a valuable educational resource.

ATTRIBUTES OF SUCCESSFUL CE METHODS

Health professionals face contextual influences when attempting to apply learning in the workplace. Processes, systems, and traditions can facilitate a learner's use of new knowledge in practice. Thus, support for change, resources, and opportunity to apply learning can both positively and negatively affect a learner's application of new knowledge (Ottoson and Patterson, 2000). While practice context can affect educational outcomes, so can the ways in which CE is delivered. The committee determined that effective CE activities have the following features:

- Incorporate needs assessments to ensure that the activity is controlled by and meets the needs of health professionals;
- Be interactive (e.g., group reflection, opportunities to practice behaviors);
- Employ ongoing feedback to engage health professionals in the learning process;
- Use multiple methods of learning and provide adequate time to digest and incorporate knowledge; and
- Simulate the clinical setting.

The foundations of these attributes are contained in bodies of theory that explain how and why CE fosters behavior that causes health professionals to evaluate their existing knowledge base when faced with clinical questions. These attributes indicate ways in which CE providers can best affect the learning of health professionals and explain, for example, why effective methods (e.g., reminders, academic detailing) tend to be more active and are used as part of a multimethod approach. The attributes provide credence to the provision of reinforcement through techniques such as audit and feedback, because these methods may motivate health professionals to change clinical behavior if their behavior is not aligned with best practices or the behavior of peers (Eisenberg, 1986; Greco and Eisenberg, 1993).

Professionals themselves, however, are primarily responsible for being self-directed, lifelong learners. They must take personal responsibility for developing their own short- and long-term learning goals and using the best available evidence to address clinical questions. Health professionals give a number of reasons for not engaging in learning outside of required CE, including lack of time, insufficient compensation (e.g., money, CE credits), or poor system support. Some health professionals see little reason to engage in self-directed learning because they believe themselves to be experts by virtue of their titles. To counteract this tendency, health care organizations and CE providers could foster a culture in which health professionals do not always feel satisfied by their current performance and understand the need for additional, advanced learning (Bierema, 2003).

CONCLUSION

The literature review of concepts that span academic disciplines provides evidence that some methods of CE—including some traditional, formal methods; informal methods; and newer, innovative methods—can be conduits for positive change in health professionals' practice. There also is evidence that health professionals often need multiple learning opportunities and multiple methods of education, such as practicing self-reflection in the workplace, reading journal articles that report new clinical evidence, and participating in formal CE lectures, if they are to most effectively change their performance and, in turn, improve patient outcomes.

The evidence is also strong, however, that continuing education is too often disconnected from theories of how adults learn and from the actual delivery of patient care. As a result, CE in its present form fails to deliver the most useful and important information to health professionals, leaving them unable to adopt evidence-based approaches efficiently to best improve patient outcomes and population health. Closing the gap will require defining research problems (Geiselman, 1984), using rigorous research techniques (Felch, 1993), developing "scholarly practitioners" (Fox, 1995, p. 5), and researching results relevant to practitioners (Conway and Clancy, 2009).

A comprehensive research agenda should do the following:

- *Identify theoretical frameworks.* Despite repeated calls for moving toward evidence-based CE (Davis et al., 1992, 1995; Mazmanian and Davis, 2002), appropriate theoretical frameworks have yet to be fully identified and tested.
- *Determine proven and innovative CE methods and the degree to which they apply in various contexts.* The literature does not conclusively identify the most effective CE delivery methods, the correct mixture of CE methods, or the amount of CE needed to maintain competency and improve clinical outcomes. CE providers have little evidence base for adopting proven and innovative methods of CE, and health professionals do not have a dependable basis for choosing one CE method over another.
- *Define CE outcome measures.* Educational theory emphasizes that effective learning requires matching the curriculum to desired outcomes. While CE aims to improve competence and thus close the gap between evidence and practice, outcomes of CE (i.e., what CE methods should explicitly aim to achieve) have not been defined for or by CE regulators, providers, or consumers. This complicates the ability of regulatory bodies to hold CE providers accountable.
- *Determine influences on learning.* The committee identified the following attributes and principles essential to the effectiveness of a CE method: needs assessments should guide CE, CE should be interactive, ongoing feedback should be employed, and CE should employ multiple learning methods. More research is needed to better understand how internal and external characteristics are associated with CE outcomes. This might include formal inquiry into the reflexivity of learning in professional practice.

REFERENCES

ACCME (Accreditation Council for Continuing Medical Education). 2008. *ACCME annual report data 2007.* http://www.accme.org/dir_docs/doc_upload/207fa8e2-bdbe-47f8-9b65-52477f9faade_uploaddocument.pdf (accessed January 16, 2009).

Argyris, C. 1991. Teaching smart people how to learn. *Harvard Business Review* May-June:99-109.

Bandura, A. 1977. *Social learning theory*. Englewood Cliffs, NJ: Prentice Hall.

Benner, P., and C. Tanner. 1987. Clinical judgment: How expert nurses use intuition. *American Journal of Nursing* 87(1):23-31.

Bennett, N. L., D. A. Davis, W. E. J. Easterling, P. Friedmann, J. S. Green, B. M. Koeppen, P. E. Mazmanian, and H. S. Waxman. 2000. Continuing medical education: A new vision of the professional development of physicians. *Academic Medicine* 75:1167-1172.

Bertram, D. A., and P. A. Brooks-Bertram. 1977. The evaluation of continuing medical education: A literature review. *Health Education Monographs* 5:330-362.

Berwick, D. 2004. *Escape fire: Designs for the future of health care*. San Francisco, CA: Jossey-Bass.

Bierema, L. L. 2003. Systems thinking: A new lens for old problems. *Journal of Continuing Education in the Health Professions* 23(S1):S27-S33.

Brookfield, S. D. 1995. *Becoming a critically reflective teacher*. San Francisco, CA: Jossey-Bass.

Bryant, S. L., T. Ringrose, and S. L. Bryant. 2005. Evaluating the doctors.net.uk model of electronic continuing medical education. *Work Based Learning in Primary Care* 3:129-142.

Carney, P. 2000. Adult learning styles: Implications for practice teaching in social work. *Social Work Education* 19(6):609-626.

Cervero, R. M. 1988. *Effective continuing education for professionals*. San Francisco, CA: Jossey-Bass.

———. 2001. Continuing professional education in transition, 1981-2000. *International Journal of Lifelong Education* 20(1-2):16-30.

Conway, P. H., and C. Clancy. 2009. Transformation of health care at the front line. *Journal of the American Medical Association* 301(7):763-765.

Cook, D. A., A. J. Levinson, S. Garside, D. M. Dupras, P. J. Erwin, and V. M. Montori. 2008. Internet-based learning in the health professions: A meta-analysis. *Journal of the American Medical Association* 300(10):1181-1196.

Cooke, M., D. M. Irby, W. Sullivan, and K. M. Ludmerer. 2006. American medical education 100 years after the Flexner report. *New England Journal of Medicine* 355(13):1339-1344.

Curry, L., and I. E. Purkis. 1986. Validity of self-reports of behavior changes by participants after a CME course. *Journal of Medical Education* 61:579-584.

Davis, B. 2004. *Inventions of teaching: A genealogy*. Mahwah, NJ: Lawrence Erlbaum.

Davis, B., and E. Simmt. 2003. Understanding learning systems: Mathematics education and complexity science. *Journal for Research in Mathematics Education* 34:137-167.

Davis, B., and D. Sumara. 2006. *Complexity and education*. Mahwah, NJ: Lawrence Erlbaum.

Davis, D., and R. D. Fox. 1994. *The physician as learner: Linking research to practice*. Chicago, IL: American Medical Association.

Davis, D., and R. Galbraith. 2009. Continuing medical education effect on practice performance: Effectiveness of continuing medical education: American College of Chest Physicians evidence-based educational guidelines. *Chest* 135(3 Suppl):42S-48S.

Davis, D. A., M. A. Thomson, A. D. Oxman, and R. B. Haynes. 1992. Evidence for the effectiveness of CME: A review of 50 randomized controlled trials. *Journal of the American Medical Association* 268(9):1111-1117.

———. 1995. Changing physician performance: A systematic review of the effect of continuing medical education strategies. *Journal of the American Medical Association* 274(9):700-705.

Davis, D., M. A. O'Brien, N. Freemantle, F. M. Wolf, P. Mazmanian, and A. Taylor-Vaisey. 1999. Impact of formal continuing medical education: Do conferences, workshops, rounds, and other traditional continuing education activities change physician behavior or health care outcomes? *Journal of the American Medical Association* 282(9):867-874.

Davis, D. A., P. E. Mazmanian, M. Fordis, R. Van Harrison, K. E. Thorpe, and L. Perrier. 2006. Accuracy of physician self-assessment compared with observed measures of competence: A systematic review. *Journal of the American Medical Association* 296(9):1094-1102.

Dennison, B., and B. Kirk. 1990. *Do, review, learn, apply: A simple guide to experience-based learning.* Oxford, UK: Blackwell.

Dixon, J. 1978. Evaluation criteria in studies of continuing education in the health professions: A critical review and a suggested strategy. *Evaluation and the Health Professions* 1(2):47-65.

Doll, W. 1993. *A post-modern perspective on curriculum.* New York: Teachers College Press.

Ebell, M. H., and A. Shaughnessy. 2003. Information mastery: Integrating continuing medical education with the information needs of clinicians. *Journal of Continuing Education in the Health Professions* 23(S1):S53-S62.

Eisenberg, J. M. 1986. *Doctors' decisions and the cost of medical care.* Ann Arbor, MI: Health Administration Press.

Eraut, M. 1994. *Developing professional knowledge and competence.* London: Falmer.

———. 2001. Do continuing professional development models promote one-dimensional learning? *Medical Education* 35(1):8-11.

Eva, K. W., and G. Regehr. 2008. "I'll never play professional football" and other fallacies of self-assessment. *Journal of Continuing Education in the Health Professions* 28(1):14-19.

Eva, K. W., J. P. Cunnington, H. I. Reiter, D. R. Keane, and G. R. Norman. 2004. How can I know what I don't know? Poor self assessment in a well-defined domain. *Advances in Health Sciences Education* 9:211-224.

Felch, W. C. 1993. Plus ça change. *Journal of Continuing Education in the Health Professions* 13(4):315-316.

Fordis, M., J. E. King, C. M. Ballantyne, P. H. Jones, K. H. Schneider, S. J. Spann, S. B. Greenberg, and A. J. Greisinger. 2005. Comparison of the instructional efficacy of Internet-based CME with live interactive CME workshops: A randomized controlled trial. *Journal of the American Medical Association* 294(9):1043-1051.

Forsetlund, L., A. Bjørndal, A. Rashidian, G. Jamtvedt, M. A. O'Brien, F. Wolf, D. Davis, J. Odgaard-Jensen, and A. D. Oxman. 2009. Continuing education meetings and workshops: Effects on professional practice and health care outcomes. *Cochrane Database Systematic Reviews*(2):CD003030.

Fox, R. D. 1995. Narrowing the gap between research and practice. *Journal of Continuing Education in the Health Professions* 15(1):1-7.

———. 2000. Using theory and research to shape the practice of continuing professional development. *Journal of Continuing Education in the Health Professions* 20:238-246.

Fox, R. D., and C. Miner. 1999. Motivation and the facilitation of change, learning, and participation in educational programs for health professionals. *Journal of Continuing Education in the Health Professions* 19(3):132-141.

Fox, R. D., P. E. Mazmanian, and R. W. Putnam, eds. 1989. *Changing and learning in the lives of physicians*. New York: Praeger.

Geiselman, L. A. 1984. Editorial. *Möbius: A Journal for Continuing Education Professionals in Health Sciences* 4(4):1-5.

Gibbs, G. 1988. *Learning by doing: A guide to teaching and learning methods*. London, UK: Federation of Entertainment Unions.

Gordon, M. J. 1991. A review of the validity and accuracy of self-assessments in health professions training. *Academic Medicine* 66(12):762-769.

Greco, P. J., and J. M. Eisenberg. 1993. Changing physicians' practices. *New England Journal of Medicine* 329:1271-1275.

Grimshaw, J. M., M. P. Eccles, A. E. Walker, and R. E. Thomas. 2002. Changing physician's behavior: What works and thoughts on getting more things to work. *Journal of Continuing Education in the Health Professions* 22(4):237-243.

Griscti, O., and J. Jacono. 2006. Effectiveness of continuing education programmes in nursing: Literature review. *Journal of Advanced Nursing* 55(4):8.

Grol, R. 2002. Changing physicians' competence and performance: Finding the balance between the individual and the organization. *Journal of Continuing Education in the Health Professions* 22(4):244-251.

Grol, R., and J. Grimshaw. 2003. From best evidence to best practice: Effective implementation of change in patient's care. *Lancet* 362(9391):1225-1230.

Harden, R. M. 2005. A new vision for distance learning and continuing medical education. *Journal of Continuing Education in the Health Professions* 25(1):43-51.

Hartzell, J. 2007. Adult learning theory in medical education. *American Journal of Medicine* 120(11):e11.

Hill, D. E. 1976. Teachers' adaptation: "Reading" and "flexing" to students. *Journal of Teacher Education* 27:268-275.

Houle, C. O. 1980. *Continuing learning in the professions*. San Francisco, CA: Jossey-Bass.

———. 1984. *Patterns of learning*. San Francisco, CA: Jossey-Bass.

IOM (Institute of Medicine). 2001. *Improving the quality of long-term care*. Washington, DC: National Academy Press.

———. 2003. *Health professions education: A bridge to quality*. Washington, DC: The National Academies Press.

Jianfei, G., S. Tregonning, and L. Keenan. 2008. Social interaction and participation: Formative evaluation of online CME modules. *Journal of Continuing Education in the Health Professions* 28(3):172-179.

Jordan, S. 2000. Educational input and patient outcomes: Exploring the gap. *Journal of Advanced Nursing* 31(2):461-471.

King, P. M., and K. S. Kitchener. 1994. *Developing reflective judgment*. San Francisco, CA: Jossey-Bass.

Knowles, M. S. 1975. *Self-directed learning: A guide for learners and teachers*. Englewood Cliffs, NJ: Prentice Hall.

———. 1980. *The modern practice of adult education. Andragogy versus pedagogy*. Englewood Cliffs, NJ: Prentice Hall/Cambridge.

Knox, A. B. 1990. Influences on participation in continuing education. *Journal of Continuing Education in the Health Professions* 10(3):261-274.

Kolb, D. A. 1984. *Experiential learning: Experience as the source of learning and development*. Englewood Cliffs, NJ: Prentice Hall.

Kues, J., D. Davis, L. Colburn, M. Fordis, I. Silver, and O. Umuhoza. 2009. *Academic CME in North America: The 2008 AAMC/SACME Harrison Survey*. Washington, DC: Association of American Medical Colleges.

Landers, M. R., J. W. McWhorter, L. L. Krum, and D. Glovinsky. 2005. Mandatory continuing education in physical therapy: Survey of physical therapists in states with and states without a mandate. *Physical Therapy* 85(9):861-871.

Long, H. B., ed. 1997. *Expanding horizons in self-directed learning*. Norman, OK: Public Managers Center, College of Education, University of Oklahoma.

MacIntosh-Murray, A., L. Perrier, and D. Davis. 2006. Research to practice in the Journal of Continuing Education in the Health Professions: A thematic analysis of volumes 1 through 24. *Journal of Continuing Education in the Health Professions* 26(3):230-243.

Maio, V., D. Belazi, N. I. Goldfarb, A. L. Phillips, and A. G. Crawford. 2003. Use and effectiveness of pharmacy continuing-education materials. *American Journal of Health-System Pharmacy* 60(16):1644-1649.

Mann, K., and J. Ribble, eds. 1994. *The role of motivation in self-directed learning*. In *The physician as learner*. Edited by D. A. Davis and R. D. Fox. Chicago, IL: American Medical Association.

Mann, K., J. Gordon, and A. MacLeod. 2007. Reflection and reflective practice in health professions education: A systematic review. *Advances in Health Sciences Education* 1-27.

Mansouri, M., and J. Lockyer. 2007. A meta-analysis of continuing medical education effectiveness. *Journal of Continuing Education in the Health Professions* 27(1):6-15.

Marinopoulos, S. S., T. Dorman, N. Ratanawongsa, L. M. Wilson, B. H. Ashar, J. L. Magaziner, R. G. Miller, P. A. Thomas, G. P. Prokopowicz, R. Qayyum, and E. B. Bass. 2007. *Effectiveness of continuing medical education*. Evidence report/technology assessment no. 149. Rockville, MD: Agency for Healthcare Research and Quality.

Mazmanian, P. E., and D. A. Davis. 2002. Continuing medical education and the physician as a learner: Guide to the evidence. *Journal of the American Medical Association* 288(9):1057-1060.

Mazmanian, P. E., D. E. Moore, R. M. Mansfield, and M. P. Neal. 1979. Perspectives on mandatory continuing medical education. *Southern Medical Journal* 72(4):378-380.

Mazmanian, P. E., D. A. Davis, and R. Galbraith. 2009. Continuing medical education effect on clinical outcomes. *Chest* 135(3 Suppl):49S-55S.

McMurtry, A. 2008. Complexity theory 101 for educators: A fictional account of a graduate seminar. *McGill Journal of Education* 43(3):265-282.

Merriam, S. B. 1987. Adult learning and theory building: A review. *Adult Education Quarterly* 37(4):187-198.

Merriam, S. B., and R. S. Caffarella. 2007. *Learning in adulthood: A comprehensive guide*. San Francisco, CA: Jossey-Bass.

Mezirow, J. 1990. *Fostering critical reflection in adulthood*. San Francisco, CA: Jossey-Bass.

Miller, G. E. 1967. Continuing education for what? *Medical Education* 42(4):320-326.

———. 1990. The assessment of clinical skills/competence/performance. *Academic Medicine* 65(9 Suppl):S63-S67.

Moon, J. 2004. Using reflective learning to improve the impact of short courses and workshops. *Journal of Continuing Education in the Health Professions* 24(1):4-11.

Moore, D. E. 2007. How physicians learn and how to design learning experiences for them: An approach based on an interpretive review of evidence. In *Continuing education in the health professions: Improving healthcare through lifelong learning*. Edited by M. Hager, S. Russell, and S. W. Fletcher. New York: Josiah Macy, Jr. Foundation.

Moore, D. E., and F. C. Pennington. 2003. Practice-based learning and improvement. *Journal of Continuing Education in the Health Professions* 23(Suppl 1):S73-S80.

Moore, D. E., J. S. Green, and H. A. Gallis. 2009. Achieving desired results and improved outcomes: Integrating planning and assessment throughout learning activities. *Journal of Continuing Education in the Health Professions* 29(1):1-15.

Nowlen, P. M. 1988. *A new approach to continuing education for business and the professions: The performance model.* New York: Macmillan.

O'Brien, M. A., N. Freemantle, A. D. Oxman, F. Wolf, D. A. Davis, and J. Herrin. 2001. Continuing education meetings and workshops: Effects on professional practice and health care outcomes. *Cochrane Database of Systematic Reviews* (online) (2).

Olson, C. A., T. R. Tooman, and J. C. Leist. 2005. Contents of a core library in continuing medical education: A Delphi study. *Journal of Continuing Education in the Health Professions* 25(4):278-288.

Osberg, D. 2005. Redescribing "education" in complex terms. *Complicity: An International Journal of Complexity and Education* 2(1):81-83.

Ottoson, J. M., and I. Patterson. 2000. Contextual influences on learning application in practice: An extended role for process evaluation. *Evaluation & the Health Professions* 23(2):194-211.

Parker III, F. W., and P. E. Mazmanian. 1992. Commitments, learning contracts, and seminars in hospital-based CME: Change in knowledge and behavior. *Journal of Continuing Education in the Health Professions* 12(1):49-63.

Pereles, L., J. Lockyer, D. Hogan, T. Gondocz, and J. Parboosingh. 1997. Effectiveness of commitment contracts in facilitating change in continuing medical education intervention. *Journal of Continuing Education in the Health Professions* 17(1):27-31.

Pew Taskforce on Health Care Workforce Regulation. 1995. *Reforming healthcare workforce regulation: Policy considerations for the 21st century.* San Francisco, CA: Pew Health Professions Commission.

Pinney, S., S. Mehta, D. Pratt, J. Sarwark, E. Campion, L. Blakemore, and K. Black. 2007. Orthopaedic surgeons as educators applying principles of adult education to teaching orthopaedic residents. *Journal of Bone and Joint Surgery* 89.

Pololi, L., M. Clay, M. Lipkin, M. Hewson, C. Kaplan, and R. Frankel. 2001. Reflections on integrating theories of adult education into a medical school faculty development course. *Medical Teacher* 23(3):276-283.

Pui, M. V., L. Liu, and S. Warren. 2005. Continuing professional education and the Internet: Views of Alberta occupational therapists. *Canadian Journal of Occupational Therapy* 72(4):234-244.

Regehr, G., and G. R. Norman. 1996. Issues in cognitive psychology: Implications for professional education. *Academic Medicine* 71(9):988-1001.

Robertson, M. K., K. E. Umble, and R. M. Cervero. 2003. Impact studies in continuing education for health professions: Update. *Journal of Continuing Education in the Health Professions* 23(3):146-156.

Sargeant, J., V. Curran, M. Allen, S. Jarvis-Selinger, and K. Ho. 2006. Facilitating interpersonal interaction and learning online: Linking theory and practice. *Journal of Continuing Education in the Health Professions* 26(2):128-136.

Schön, D. 1983. *The reflective practitioner: How professionals think in action.* New York: Basic Books.

———. 1987. *Educating the reflective practitioner.* San Francisco, CA: Jossey-Bass.

Segrave, S., and D. Holt. 2003. Contemporary learning environments: Designing e-learning for education in the professions. *Distance Education* 24(1):7-24.

Sibley, J. C., D. L. Sackett, V. Neufeld, B. Gerrard, K. V. Rudnick, and W. Fraser. 1982. A randomized trial of continuing medical education. *New England Journal of Medicine* 306(9):511-515.

Slotnick, H. B., and M. B. Shershneva. 2002. Use of theory to interpret elements of change. *Journal of Continuing Education in the Health Professions* 22(4):197-204.

Smith, C. A., A. Cohen-Callow, D. A. Dia, D. L. Bliss, A. Gantt, L. J. Cornelius, and D. Harrington. 2006. Staying current in a changing profession: Evaluating perceived change resulting from continuing professional education. *Journal of Social Work Education* 42(3):465-482.

Smith, M. K. 2001. *Donald Schön: Learning, reflection and change.* http://www.infed.org/thinkers/et-schon.htm (accessed March 4, 2009).

Stanton, F., and J. Grant. 1999. Approaches to experiential learning, course delivery and validation in medicine. A background document. *Medical Education* 33(4):282-297.

Stein, L. S. 1981. The effectiveness of continuing medical education: Eight research reports. *Journal of Medical Education* 56(2):103-110.

Tian, J., N. L. Atkinson, B. Portnoy, and R. S. Gold. 2007. A systematic review of evaluation in formal continuing medical education. *Journal of Continuing Education in the Health Professions* 27(1):16-27.

Tough, A. 1971. *The adult's learning projects: A fresh approach to theory and practice of adult learning.* Toronto: Ontario Institute for Studies in Education.

U.S. Department of Health, Education, and Welfare. 1967. *Report of the National Advisory Committee on Health Manpower.* Washington, DC: U.S. Government Printing Office.

Wakefield, A. B., C. Carlisle, A. G. Hall, and M. J. Attree. 2008. The expectations and experiences of blended learning approaches to patient safety education. *Nurse Education in Practice* 8(1):54-61.

Wakefield, J., C. P. Herbert, M. Maclure, C. Dormuth, J. M. Wright, J. Legare, P. Brett-MacLean, and J. Premi. 2003. Commitment to change statements can predict actual change in practice. *Journal of Continuing Education in the Health Professions* 23(2):81-93.

Wensing, M., H. Wollersheim, and R. Grol. 2006. Organizational interventions to implement improvements in patient care: A structured review of reviews. *Implementation Science* 1(1):1-9.

Wutoh, R., S. A. Boren, and E. A. Balas. 2004. E-learning: A review of Internet-based continuing medical education. *Journal of Continuing Education in the Health Professions* 24(1):20-30.

3

Regulation and Financing

Regulation and financing are critical components of continuing education (CE). The regulation of CE is arguably intended to be a proxy for quality, as it establishes a minimum set of quality standards, while the financing pays for the conduct and research of CE activities. However, regulatory and financing mechanisms for CE are disconnected from and poorly aligned with the goals of improving health professionals' performance. Little uniformity exists in CE regulation and financing across health professions, inhibiting development of a modern, integrated, team-oriented workforce. This chapter explores regulation and financing of continuing education in the largest sectors of the health care workforce—medicine, nursing, pharmacy, and social work.[1]

REGULATION OF CONTINUING EDUCATION IN SELECT HEALTH PROFESSIONS

The current regulation of CE attempts to ensure high quality learning for health professionals by targeting individual professionals through licensure, certification, and credentialing, and by targeting providers of learning activities through accreditation. As

---

[1] These are the largest professions as measured by numbers of professionals, with more than 200,000 clinicians. The committee recognizes the various health professions identified in Appendix B but was unable to describe each profession in depth.

is the case with most other aspects of health care, each profession approaches regulation differently, using variable terminology and approaches to CE, employing different learning requirements, and developing unique regulatory processes.

Regulating Individual Health Professionals

Since the early 1970s, CE for health professionals has been linked directly to licensure, certification, and credentialing. The various regulatory authorities—states for licensure, specialty societies for certification, and health care organizations for credentialing—attempt to ensure that a given health professional's background meets some minimal standard of quality.

Learning tools such as self-assessment, peer evaluation, and learning portfolios should all have a role in supporting the acquisition of knowledge and skills, reinforcing competence, and reassuring the public's trust (Cooke et al., 2006). However, current licensing and certification systems principally assess learning only by measuring health professionals' participation in CE. Despite some professions' efforts to recognize achievement in knowledge, competence, and performance (Miller et al., 2008), the systems are still strongly linked to participation and not specifically focused on measures that really matter—changes in professional behavior and patient outcomes.

Licensure

In many health professions, professionals are mandated by law to receive a license to practice from a state licensing board (Mazmanian et al., 1979), and health professionals may hold a license in more than one state. This requirement is arguably the strongest regulatory tool available to assess individual health professionals. However, licensure has been linked only tangentially to performance improvement (Davis et al., 2003). Moreover, while initial licensure establishes the minimum competence required for admission to a profession, it does not guarantee that a health professional will maintain competency or provide a high level of care.

Many states call for health professionals to apply for periodic relicensure, which often requires varying amounts of CE credits or hours. Requirements differ greatly by state and by health profession (see Figure 3-1). The various professional state boards are represented by national organizations, such as the Federation of State Medical Boards and the National Council of State Boards of Nursing. CE licensure requirements are generally organized around

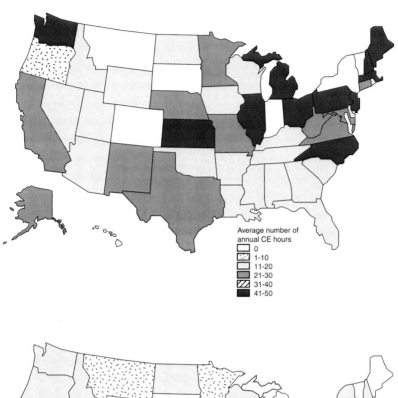

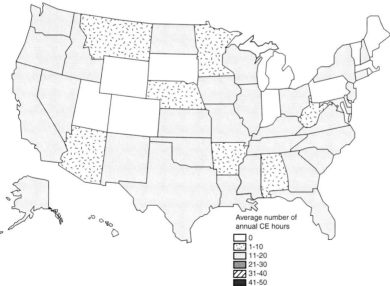

FIGURE 3-1 Average number of annual CE hours for physicians (M.D.s) (top) compared with physical therapists (bottom).

TABLE 3-1 Examples of CME Activities by Category

Category 1	Category 2
Publishing articles	Consultation with peers
Poster presentations	Small-group discussion
Medically related advanced degrees	Self-assessment activities
Independent learning	Medical writing
Live or attendance-based activities	Teaching residents
Journal reading[a]	

[a] Journal reading is counted for Category 1 credit only when providers (i.e., journals) incorporate mechanisms for reflection and/or interaction with the article content. This requirement can be met through an evaluation or examination that physicians return to the provider.

learning activities that often are conducted in groups, such as at conferences and lectures, and the content and processes of learning are under the control of the CE provider. Licensure has been linked only tangentially to performance improvement (Davis et al., 2003).

Often, licensure and relicensure require certain amounts of particular types of CE activities, which are divided into "formal" and "informal" categories. For example, in medicine, these categories refer to Category 1 and Category 2™, defined and trademarked by the American Medical Association (2006) (see Table 3-1). To meet continuing medical education (CME) licensure and relicensure requirements, physicians must participate in a specified number of Category 1 and Category 2 activities, but only Category 1 activities count toward the required number of credits. The relative benefit of Category 1 over Category 2 activities is questionable, however, because some learning methods appear more effective than others, as discussed in Chapter 2. For example, self-assessment, a Category 2 activity, often imparts more lasting knowledge retention than a lecture, a Category 1 activity. Thus, the typical emphasis placed on providing and obtaining Category 1 credits may divert limited resources from more effective Category 2 activities.

Certification

Certification is the process by which professional specialty societies or credentialing bodies—not regulatory bodies—certify individual health professionals as qualified experts to practice in a particular area of a profession. In professions that require certification, such as medicine (under specialty boards), professionals must regularly repeat the certification processes, which differ by profession and by specialty. The American Board of Medical Specialties has recently adopted new standards for a four-component mandatory maintenance-of-certification program: the components focus on professional standing, lifelong learning and self-assessment, cognitive expertise, and evaluation of performance in practice. Instead of recertification being required once every 10 years, this shift toward a new type of maintenance of certification requires continual engagement in professional development (ABMS, 2009).

Credentialing

Credentialing occurs at the level of health care organizations, such as hospitals and group practices, that employ health professionals. Organizations use credentialing in an attempt to ensure that health professionals are qualified to practice and maintain a minimum level of competence and performance. Many organizations use credentialing as the basis for granting staff privileges, and some organizations also credential health professionals for particular procedures, based on their experience and clinical outcomes. Many organizations develop their own credentialing guidelines. The process can be likened to an audit. Credentialing often includes, at a minimum, review and verification of a health professional's licensure, education, and certification, if applicable.

Examples of Fragmentation in Select Health Professions

The variation in the numbers of required CE credits (see Figure 3-1) and the content of such learning exemplifies the fragmentation in the current state of CE (see Table 3-2). Among the problems that such variation causes, current CE does not generally promote team-based learning. For example, health professionals do not normally learn with clinicians from other professions, partially as a result of disconnected and dissimilar CE systems. Health professionals from one profession also typically cannot earn CE credit for attending an activity offered by another profession, regardless of the degree to which the content may overlap and the relationships may foster collaborative practice.

Regulatory variations also result in some types of health professionals receiving more continuing education than others. For example, nurses are required to take only 5 hours of CE annually in one state and 15 hours in others. The picture is similar for pharmacists; some states require them to receive 10-60 credits per year to remain licensed, while some states have no CE requirements. In other pro-

TABLE 3-2 Comparison of CE Providers, Activities, Requirements, and Consequences of Failing to Meet Those Requirements in Four Health Professions

Health Profession	Types of CE Providers
Medicine	• Hospitals or health care delivery systems • Insurance or managed care organizations • Nonprofit foundations • Physician membership organizations • Specialty organizations • Publishing/education companies • Schools of medicine • State medical societies
Nursing	• Government organizations • Hospital or health delivery systems • Publishing/education companies • Schools of nursing • State nursing associations • Nursing specialty organizations
Pharmacy	• Colleges or schools of pharmacy • Publishing/education companies • Pharmaceutical manufacturers • Pharmacy professional organizations or associations • Government agencies • Hospitals or health delivery networks
Social Work	• Nonprofit organizations • Publishing/education companies • Social work professional societies and associations • Schools of social work • Government organizations • Web-based companies

[a] Range is given for jurisdictions that require CE, because some states do not require CE in all professions.

[b] Activities include seminars, workshops, teaching activities, course preparation, web-based courses, self-study experiences, and professional publication.

fessions, some states require that CE credits be taken in specific areas, such as HIV/AIDS and domestic violence, according to the profession. Certification requirements also differ by individual specialty boards. Increasingly, hospitals, insurers, and even partners in clinical practice require varying amounts and types of CE activities (Peck, 2000).

Examples of Accredited CE Activities	CE Required per Year[a]	Repercussions for Failing to Receive CE
• Live activities • Learning procedures • Enduring materials • Performance improvement • Journal-based continuing medical education (CME) • Manuscript review • Test-item writing • Web-based point-of-care learning	10-75 CME credits	• Loss of licensure or credentialing • Loss of membership in professional organizations • Loss of membership in provider organizations, higher medical liability premiums, fines
• Educational meetings • Lectures • Courses • Approved review materials • Computer- and web-based courses	5-15 contact hours	• License suspension or revocation • Report to national data banks • Fines
• Knowledge-based continuing professional education (CPE) to acquire factual knowledge • Application-based CPE to apply knowledge learned • Practice-based CPE	10-60 CPE hours	• Disciplinary actions against one's pharmacy license • Further CPE requirements • Fines
• Formally organized learning events[b] • Professional meetings or organized learning experiences • Individual professional activities	3-25 CE hours	• Withholding licensure

Regulation in social work is particularly variable; for example, states differ greatly in how they establish licensure categories and what titles they confer. Various licenses (e.g., licensed clinical social worker, licensed social worker, licensed graduate social worker) can be accompanied by vastly different requirements. Among states that mandate CE for licensure of social workers, requirements range from 9 hours every 3 years to 50 hours every 2 years. While state board requirements vary, the National Association of Social Workers (NASW, 2003) has developed a separate, voluntary set of standards for CE that requires social workers to complete 48 hours of CE every 2 years to be recognized at the national level.

If health professionals fail to fulfill CE requirements, various degrees of repercussions and disciplinary action occur. Generally, health professionals are fined or suspended, and they may face revocation of licensure or credentialing, higher medical liability premiums, or loss of membership in professional and provider organizations. In nursing and other professions, a lapse in CE participation may be reported to state and federal data banks.

Many state boards conduct random audits of individual professionals to verify that they indeed completed their required CE activities. The Oregon State Board of Nursing, for example, audits a certain percentage of applicants for relicensure each month by requesting copies of CE certificates of completion (Grossman, 1998), and many state medical boards audit 1-25 percent of physicians per year to check whether they completed required CME activities (AMA, 2008).

However, not all health professions require ongoing licensure, certification, or credentialing. Many allied health professions' professional competency requirements are minimal beyond initial licensure and certification, and professionals are not required to relicense or recertify. For example, until recently, a licensed physical therapist was "entitled to practice indefinitely" (Brosky and Scott, 2007). Defining, assessing, and measuring ongoing professional competence in physical therapy has recently garnered attention, as the profession has become more autonomous (as exemplified by direct access to patients without a referral) and the doctor of physical therapy has become the entry-level degree.

Consistent Licensure, Certification, and Credentialing

Licensure, certification, and credentialing need to become more consistent, and standardized requirements need to be established, to help ensure minimal levels of competence. Efforts to align these processes have begun to occur in small pockets. For example, the nursing community is moving toward greater unanimity around CE requirements for licensure across states. Therefore, licensure, certification, and credentialing ought to reward improvement of competence, performance, and patient health, instead of focusing merely on rewarding skills, as is now the case.

It will be important for the regulatory system to recognize the inextricable linkage between the continuing education of all health care professionals and health care teams, the quality of patient care, and the quality of system performance. This will require developing linkages among the various regulators of health care and developing new standards and processes. Today's simple credit system, which reinforces the isolated "silo" structure that characterizes regulatory activities, should be abandoned. The organizations involved in regulation should work together to define the purposes of regulations and the areas on which regulators should focus. Standards should be developed that attend to the linkages in ways that reinforce the work of each regulatory system. Action needs to be taken to foster and publicly recognize team-based, local, and national learning about good regulation and good health care.

Licensure and certification processes should reward successful demonstration of maintenance of competence. Additionally, certification should require a minimum standard of practice-based learning to promote the identification and solution of practice-based needs. To promote reflection, licensure or credentialing should require demonstrated use of learning portfolios with documented needs assessments. Learning activities should be granted licensure or credentialing only if they have demonstrated effectiveness for improving professionals' learning or performance, or for improving patient outcomes.

Accreditation of CE Providers in Select Health Professions

Accredited CE providers include organizations such as hospital systems, professional membership and specialty organizations, publishing/education companies, professional schools, and, in some cases, state boards. Accreditation bodies generally conduct formal accreditation processes at both regional and national levels. Accreditation attempts to confirm the quality and integrity of accredited CE by establishing criteria for the evaluation of the providers, assessing whether accredited providers meet and maintain minimum standards, and promoting provider self-assessment and improvement (Michigan State Medical Society Committee on CME Accreditation, 2009). Accreditation bodies evolved as an effort to assure the professions and the public of the quality of teaching and education in the health professions. Box 3-1 provides an example of the development of the Accreditation Council for Continuing Medical Education (ACCME).

BOX 3-1
History: Development of the ACCME

Continuing medical education (CME) in the United States includes a long history of American Medical Association (AMA) initiatives to acknowledge physicians' participation in CME and to approve state medical societies as accreditors of regional CME programs. In 1968, the AMA developed the Physician's Recognition Award (AMA/PRA), which is awarded to physicians who participate in 150 hours or more of CME during a 3-year period. In 1971, the AMA decided that only courses offered by organizations accredited by the AMA Council on Medical Education would count toward the award.

As demands grew to make participation in CME mandatory for medical relicensure, professional society memberships, specialty certification, and credentialing, the AMA Council on Medical Education delegated select accreditation tasks to local or regional organizations, including state medical societies. In 1977, the AMA helped to initiate the Liaison Committee on Continuing Medical Education (LCCME), which assumed the accreditation role previously held by the AMA Council on Medical Education. The LCCME and its successor, the Accreditation Council for Continuing Medical Education (ACCME), included various participation.[a] The ACCME currently serves as the body that accredits institutions and organizations nationally to offering CME and to designating Category 1 credit, and recognizes institutions and organizations, including state medical societies, to confer CME accreditation that enables the designation of Category 1 credit for qualified CME activities.

---

[a] Participants included the AMA, American Board of Medical Specialties, American Hospital Association, Association for Hospital Medical Education, Association of American Medical Colleges, Council of Medical Specialty Societies, and Federation of State Medical Boards.

Current State of Accreditation

Depending on the profession, some accreditors review the quality of specific CE activities and programs, while others attempt to assess CE providers themselves. Entities wishing to provide CE may voluntarily pursue accreditation. In granting accreditation, accreditors look for such things as whether the CE provider provides a written mission statement reflecting the values and ethics of the profession and whether it will assist professionals in maintaining and enhancing professional competencies to practice in various settings. As an example of such efforts, the criteria used by the American Nurses Credentialing Center (ANCC) are listed in Box 3-2. Additionally, each profession has developed specific regulations regarding

BOX 3-2
Example of Accreditation Criteria

The American Nurses Credentialing Center, a major national accreditation body for continuing nursing education (CNE), defines the following criteria for provider accreditation:

- CNE must be conducted by accredited "provider units," which should document that the organizations' beliefs and goals are relevant and appropriate to prospective learners;
- CNE activities must be tailored to the educational needs of the target audience;
- Each educational activity must be planned by groups with the relevant content expertise and representation from the target audience;
- Each CNE activity must be designed with an identified purpose and learner objectives, content and teaching strategies to achieve the objectives, and criteria for completion of the CE activity; and
- Each CNE activity must include an evaluative measure that includes learner input and a method for verifying that participation in the activity occurred.

conflicts of interest and commercial support for CE activities and providers.

CE providers can apply for an accreditation period of 4-6 years in many health professions (e.g., medicine, nursing, pharmacy). The accreditation process requires ongoing evaluation and improvement processes and contact with providers. For example, in medicine, the ACCME calls on a group of more than 150 volunteers to interview providers applying for reaccreditation and requires providers to submit an annual report describing the size and scope of activities planned and executed. The ANCC conducts site visits of continuing nursing education (CNE) providers to ensure their quality; those that do not adhere to requirements can have their accreditation suspended or revoked (ANCC, 2009).

In pharmacy, pharmaceutical manufacturers directly provide continuing education, but these CE providers must plan all activities independent of commercial interests and present their materials to participants with full disclosure of manufacturer participation and sufficient balance. Social work associations in certain states also accredit CE providers; many states do not require preapproval of CE providers, but instead depend on the social workers they license to ensure that CE activities comply with state administrative requirements.

Consistent Accreditation

Establishing consistent accreditation standards across professions and states would have a number of advantages. Standardization would allow the already underresourced accreditation infrastructure to be streamlined around common procedures. It would also reduce the potential for programs that have been declined accreditation by one agency to take advantage of lenient accreditation standards elsewhere, and it would promote a system of sharing best practices, as other accreditors could apply similar standards. Standardized accreditation requirements would become the expectation of learners, allowing learners to more easily identify deviations from the norm. Consistent accreditation requirements adopted across professions would facilitate interprofessional education in CE because providers would accredit their courses for multiple types of health professionals who would learn together.

FINANCING OF CONTINUING EDUCATION[2]

Financing is an overarching issue in any discussion of CE because innovations in learning require that teachers, students, and organizations have the necessary resources for learning (Cooke et al., 2006). The financing of CE, as with its regulation, varies by profession. Table 3-3 provides an overview of CE financing in medicine.

CE Providers

Continuing education is provided by many different entities. A complete breakdown is not available for all health professions, but Figure 3-2 shows CE providers in medicine. Medical schools provide the most hours of continuing medical education (45 percent of the total). Professional societies and organizations provide nearly a quarter of all CME hours, and they also are important providers outside of medicine (ACCME, 2008). Employers of health care professionals, such as the Department of Veterans Affairs (VA), and health

---

[2] The best estimate of financing in CE available for this analysis was from the ACCME Annual Report Data, which provides information only in medicine. Therefore, this section focuses mainly on financing in medicine but may have implications for other health professions.

TABLE 3-3 Overview of Current CE Financing in Medicine

	Current System
Industry funding?	Yes, ~58% of total
Out-of-pocket cost to physicians	~42% of total, or $1,200 per physician per year
Mode of delivery	Primarily in-person lectures and workshops, with a small amount of simulation training and performance improvement exercises taking hold
Educational value, impact on patient care	Unclear

care institutions, such as hospitals and insurers, may also provide continuing education. Particularly in medicine and pharmacy, commercial CE institutions are important providers of CE.

Commercial entities include medical education and communication companies (MECCs), which are generally for-profit companies hired by commercial interests to organize meetings, find speakers for conferences or lectures, and develop enduring materials (Coogle, 2008; Steinbrook, 2005). A 2007 quantitative survey of 79 MECCs found that 53 percent reported being part of a larger organization that included companies involved in commercial promotion (Peterson et al., 2008). Even though many commercial companies are accredited by the ACCME, their motivations have sometimes been questioned due to the potential bias they introduce and the volume of CE they provide (Blumenthal, 2004; Brennan et al., 2006; DeAngelis and Fontanarosa, 2008; United States Senate Committee on Finance, 2007).

Cost of CME

Data on the costs of CE outside medicine are limited. In 2007, the total cost of CME provided at a national level was $2.54 billion, consisting of commercial support, advertising and exhibit income, and registration fees and other income. On average, ACCME providers generated profits of 23.5 percent, as shown in Table 3-4. Professional societies derived the largest profit margins (31.8 percent). Publishing/education companies, which include but are not exclu-

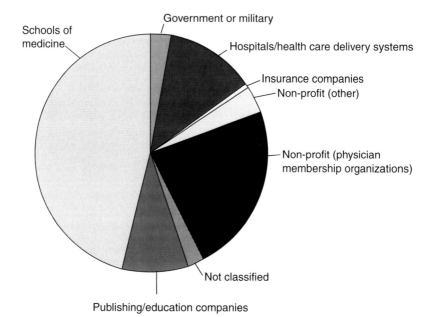

FIGURE 3-2 Hours of directly sponsored CME by organization type.
SOURCE: ACCME, 2008.

sively composed of MECCs, derived 25.9 percent profit margins
(ACCME, 2008).

Who Pays for CE?

Financing of CE varies by profession. Some health professionals
pay out of pocket for their CE, while employers, commercial entities,
and others may pay for all or part of the continued learning expenses
of other professionals. Thus, CE funding comes from numerous
sources, including health professionals themselves, employers, commercial entities, and the government.

In many health professions, including occupational therapy and
dentistry, health professionals are generally responsible for paying
for a majority of their own CE. This culture of paying out of pocket
for CE closely resembles the culture in other industries (e.g., certified
public accountants). When the costs are borne by individuals, they
are likely to choose an activity based on its perceived value, which
may, however, be based more on the activity's cost and convenience
than its content and clinical benefit. In 2007, physicians paid 42

percent ($1.05 billion) of the total $2.54 billion spent on CME. On average, a physician paid slightly more than $1,400 per year for his CME.[3] Data on the costs of CE paid by individual health professionals in each profession were unavailable for this assessment.

Some organizations see continuing education as an investment in staff development and bear at least a portion of CE costs. The opportunity costs of lost staff time, as well as the fees and other costs associated with an activity, may, however, be seen as a drain on health care organizations in times of shrinking financial resources.

The federal government provides little direct financing for CE for health professionals, especially compared with the billions of dollars of public support for graduate and undergraduate education. Public funds are used, for example, toward the CE of professionals sponsored by the VA, the Department of Defense, and the Indian Health Service. Some other federal funds support CE activities. For example, the Health Resources and Services Administration provides some funding for health professions CE through Titles VII and VIII of the Public Health Service Act. No consistent investment for a large majority of nongovernment-related health professionals exists.

Particularly in medicine and pharmacy (and nursing to a lesser extent), funding for CE also comes through direct funding of CE providers from a variety of sources, including employers, professional societies, and commercial entities.

Issues Around Funding and Provision of CE

Two current features of CE funding may inhibit achievement of better CE. One concern arises because of the role of commercial funding and the conflicts of interest that may result. A second concern is that the silo structure of many professional organizations and education institutions may inhibit learning and interprofessional collaboration.

---

[3] The total income into the CME system ($2.54 billion) was the minuend from which the total commercial support ($1.5 billion) was subtracted. The difference ($1.04 billion) was presumed by the researchers to be the amount paid out of pocket by physicians. This figure was divided by 718,000, the approximate number of active physicians (not including residents and fellows) in the United States in 2007 (personal communication, J. Cultice, Health Resources and Services Administration, May 27, 2009). The resulting figure was taken to be a rough estimate of the out-of-pocket cost per physician per year.

TABLE 3-4 Financial Support of CME for Different Types of Organizations, 2007

Organization Type	Number	Total Income	Commercial Support
Government or military	15	$69.5 million	$0.25 million (<0.5%)
Hospital or health care delivery system	93	$105 million	$47.5 million (45.2%)
Insurance company or managed care	14	$3.49 million	$0.32 million (9.2%)
Nonprofit (other)	38	$160.4 million	$78.4 million (48.9%)
Nonprofit (physician member organization)	270	$887.2 million	$215.4 million (24.3%)
Not classified	33	$55.2 million	$29.3 million (53.1%)
Publishing or education company	150	$830.8 million	$594.4 million (71.5%)
School of medicine	123	$427.7 million	$245.8 million (57.5%)
Total	736	$2.54 billion	$1.21 billion (47.7%)

SOURCE: ACCME, 2008.

Conflict of Interest

Medically related industries, such as pharmaceutical and medical device companies, have taken a lead role in financing the research on and provision of CE in medicine and pharmacy, despite much controversy (Peterson et al., 2008). Since the 1960s, the dependence of CE on commercial funds has raised concerns about bias and conflicts of interest with respect to companies using CE as a means of inappropriately influencing health professionals, especially physicians, to increase their market shares (Podolsky and Greene, 2008). The first published empirical evidence found that approximately 43 percent of CE programs for pharmacists received commercial support, and that such high levels of support helped to create a culture

Advertising and Exhibit Income	Registration Fees and Other Income	Total Expense	Profit Margin (%)
$0.38 million (0.55%)	$68.8 million (99.0%)	$69.2 million	0.4
$7.4 million (7.0%)	$50.1 million (47.7%)	$100.3 million	4.5
$0.035 million (1.0%)	$3.14 million (90.0%)	$6.72 million	−92.6
$11.9 million (7.4%)	$70.1 million (43.7%)	$126.5 million	21.1
$217.9 million (24.6%)	$453.9 million (51.2%)	$605.3 million	31.8
$2.4 million (4.3%)	$23.5 million (42.6%)	$43.7 million	20.8
$10.8 million (1.3%)	$225.6 million (27.2%)	$615.7 million	25.9
$23.2 million (5.4%)	$158.7 million (37.1)	$375.8 million	12.1
$274.0 million (10.8%)	$1.05 billion (41.5%)	$1.94 billion	23.6

in which pharmacists expect to obtain CE at a minimal cost and CE providers "are dependent on industry to assist them in covering administrative, educational, and noneducational expenses" (Smith et al., 2006, p. 310).

In 2007, $1.5 billion[4] of CME funding came from commercial entities. Some efforts have been made to develop safeguards meant to ensure that CE providers are free from conflicts of interest. Yet widespread skepticism remains as to CE funders' intentions

---

[4] The total commercial support listed in the ACCME Annual Report Data (2008) is $1.21 billion; convention also adds the amount spent on advertising and exhibits income, $275 million, to derive the more complete $1.5 billion in commercial support.

(DeAngelis and Fontanarosa, 2008; Peterson et al., 2008; Relman, 2001; Steinbrook, 2008). The Institute of Medicine (IOM) Committee on Conflict of Interest in Medical Research, Education, and Practice has addressed these issues in depth and has recommended, among other things, that industry should not influence CME (IOM, 2009).

It is important to note that MECCs and other conflicted sources[5] can be significant resources, for example, by supplying well-trained staff who provide high quality CE. Also, significant progress has been made in the past 5 years toward protecting educational content from potentially corrupting influences and promotional intent (ACCME, 2006; PhRMA, 2008). As in other health professions, the ACCME has detailed regulations to ensure that commercial interests are kept separate from learning activities and course content. The regulations require CME providers to disclose conflicts of interest and resolve relevant financial relationships with any commercial interest among those in a position to control CME content. For example, the ACCME requires CME providers to give a balanced view of therapeutic options and encourages the use of generic names of therapies, rather than promoting specific proprietary names (ACCME, 2006). Still, such efforts may not be sufficient to keep activities free from bias. For example, in some CME activities, conflicted sources are alleged to have planted members in audiences to ask specific questions about a particular drug, ensuring that the discussion will include that drug (McCartney, 2004). To monitor bias in CME, the ACCME requires providers to survey participants about potential commercial bias at the conclusion of events. Participants, however, may not necessarily be the best detectors of this bias (Steinbrook, 2005). The committee concludes that CE should be free of influence from conflicts of interest to protect the integrity of health professional development.

Interprofessional Collaboration

Although professional societies and organizations have important roles to play in continuing education, they also may be the sources of some problems. For example, their influence may be counterproductive to interprofessional collaboration, standards of certification, and patient care if they focus too narrowly on profession-specific interests and not on the best ways to improve health. Professional

---

[5] In the context of this report, conflicted sources are those that use CE primarily as a mechanism for advertising and marketing for their own personal or corporate gain and not for the continued improvement of health care quality and patient safety.

societies also may have potential conflicts of interest between their roles as protectors of the profession and providers of the learning that will drive collective competence. The roles of professional organizations need to explicitly include jointly fostering interprofessional education, promoting appropriate evidence-based approaches, and supporting lifelong learning. Checks and balances will be needed to ensure that professional societies are meeting all of these obligations appropriately.

Future Financing for a More Comprehensive System

Whether continuing education for health professionals should be financed by government, industry, employers, or individuals is still being debated. What is clear, however, is that funding should be directly aligned with the goals of driving improved quality of care and patient safety and should support a mix of activities that are effective both in terms of performance and cost. In this way, funding will help in developing a more comprehensive, broad-based system for professional development, called continuing professional development (CPD), as described in Chapter 1. In addition, strong safeguards need to be put in place to avert the development of education solely for the sake of profit, thus protecting the integrity of the system.

This shift of focus and priorities will almost certainly have implications for the amount of support available for CPD and its sources. Sources of CPD funding are unlikely to remain static because a market for CPD exists. As some sources disappear, new ones will likely emerge. To be responsive to changes in the field and the rapidly changing needs of the health professions, flexibility will be a necessary attribute of CPD funding structures.

Some commercial supporters are already looking past short-term, profit-driven CE toward funding programs that have the most impact on physician performance (Saxton, 2009). Figure 3-3 explores the intersection of areas of "business needs," "healthcare system quality gaps," "healthcare provider performance gaps," and "patient needs." This portrayal suggests that industry support could be of greatest value for all stakeholders at this intersection, if the purpose of the activity is to improve quality and patient safety. To identify the areas where industry needs and funding could align with the needs of the health care system, an effective research enterprise will have to be in place to identify gaps in the current system and to develop theories and effective interventions to fill them.

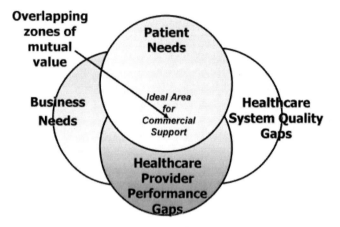

FIGURE 3-3 A convergence-of-interest model of commercial support.
SOURCE: Saxton, 2009.

The availability of industry funding has the potential to influence the types of CE programs offered. Currently, if alignment with industry interests determines the content of continuing education, areas of health care and patient safety that fall outside of industry interests generally receive less support. For example, if industry only funds therapeutics that are based in medications, these topics will be of greater priority for CE providers but may not be more effective in yielding better outcomes than other types of CE. This is inconsistent with a system of learner-driven CPD and needs to be remedied in the development of a new model of CPD funding.

One interesting question to ask is, what might happen if commercial funding were entirely withdrawn and no subsidies were provided by other sources? The average physician could fund his own CME and continue attending the same types of CME activities by investing about $3,500 annually.[6] Although this is a rough estimate and does not take into account the nuances of the various sources of CME funding, it provides a general sense of how

---

[6] The figure is calculated by dividing $2.54 billion by 718,000 physicians, the number of active physicians (not including residents or fellows) in 2007 as reported by the Health Resources and Services Administration from the American Medical Association Physician Masterfile (personal communication, J. Cultice, Health Resources and Services Administration, May 27, 2009). A recent article estimates $4,013 spent per physician in 2007, based on a denominator of 633,000 physicians, a figure reported by the U.S. Bureau of Labor Statistics for physicians and surgeons in 2006 (Mazmanian, 2009).

much CME would cost. Without funding from conflicted sources, CE content would likely shift away from knowledge about specific drugs and devices. It is not clear, though, precisely how the content would change in the event conflicted funding sources disappeared because the content and types of CE that are biased and sponsored by conflicted sources is not well-defined. Also, it is important to understand that under such circumstances, CME providers may also change the amount and types of CE activities they sponsor.

Even if CME did not change, physicians could continue to fulfill existing regulatory CME requirements without increasing their out-of-pocket spending. For example, through journals such as the *New England Journal of Medicine* and the *Journal of the American Medical Association*, a physician can fulfill Category 1 regulatory requirements by paying approximately $150-$750 for an entire year's worth of 50 credits. These examples demonstrate how regulatory requirements can be satisfied while spending less than the average physician currently spends on CME. However, it is unlikely that all physicians would choose to adopt only low-cost, convenient CME, because they would likely be motivated to network and learn in part through other methods, such as live activities. In the event a credit-based system is used, regulatory and quasi-regulatory bodies could also place restrictions on the types of CME for which physicians can receive credit, ensuring that they receive CE credits through a variety of methods tailored to the specific learning needs and contexts.

Since not all physicians would choose the lowest-cost, most convenient methods, a medium-cost CME option might assume that physicians participate in CME not only to fulfill CME requirements but also to prepare for periodic recertification exams. Exam-preparatory CME would cost approximately $550 per physician per year.[7] As in the journal-based CME option, many physicians would likely desire and choose to participate in higher quality, interactive CME events to network, update, and maintain their knowledge base. Physicians could fulfill most CME requirements by using inexpensive methods and spending less than they do now, leaving funds to attend some higher-cost, higher-value CME events. Therefore, a mix of cost-effective CE could be achievable in the current financing

---

[7] The average annual cost of recertification, calculated from the following medical specialties as of March 2009: allergy and immunology, anesthesiology, colon and rectal surgery, dermatology, emergency medicine, family medicine, internal medicine, neurological surgery, nuclear medicine, obstetrics and gynecology, ophthalmology, orthopedic surgery, pediatrics, physical medicine and rehabilitation, plastic surgery, psychiatry and neurology, radiology, surgery, thoracic surgery, and urology.

environment. However, no evidence exists to predict how physicians would respond to changes in CE financing.

In the absence of evidence, the committee assumes that physicians could maintain participation in activities similar to the ones in which they currently participate (e.g., a hybrid of low-cost, journal-based CME with occasional participation in higher quality, higher cost activities) without paying more out of pocket.

Although the question of what would happen were commercial support removed is critically important, no empirical evidence exists to date to support or refute hypotheses of how commercial supporters would respond. A determination cannot be made of whether the costs of an ideal system would be greater than the costs of the current system.

Funding is unequal and unstable across all health professions. The lack of data about the financing of CE is alarming because data are needed to determine how to invest most efficiently in CE. Current methods of financing cannot support a comprehensive, evidence-based learning system that promotes high quality, high value health care that is free from conflict of interest. It is likely, however, that sufficient funding exists within the current structure to support better learning. If better aligned with overall efforts to improve the quality of care, continuing professional development could maintain professional competence and help prepare professionals to improve patient outcomes in the absence of industry funding. Significant spending that currently supports less effective activities could and should be redirected toward more effective activities to counter the significant losses from conflicted funding sources.

REFERENCES

ABMS (American Board of Medical Specialties). 2009. *ABMS maintenance of certification.* http://abms.org/Maintenance_of_Certification/ABMS_MOC.aspx (accessed April 23, 2009).
ACCME (Accreditation Council for Continuing Medical Education). 2006. *ACCME essential areas and their elements: Updated decision-making criteria relevant to the essential areas and elements.* Chicago, IL: ACCME.
———. 2008. *ACCME annual report data 2007.* http://www.accme.org/dir_docs/doc_upload/207fa8e2-bdbe-47f8-9b65-52477f9faade_uploaddocument.pdf (accessed January 16, 2009).
AMA (American Medical Association). 2006. *The physician's recognition award and credit system: Information for accredited providers and physicians.* Edited by the American Medical Association. http://www.ama-assn.org/ama1/pub/upload/mm/455/pra2006.pdf.
———. 2008. *State medical licensure requirements and statistics, 2008.* Chicago, IL: AMA Press.

ANCC (American Nurses Credentialing Center). 2009. *ANCC accreditation application manual.* http://www.nursecredentialing.org/ContinuingEducation/Accreditation/AccreditationProcess.aspx (accessed July 15, 2009).

Blumenthal, D. 2004. Doctors and drug companies. *New England Journal of Medicine* 351(18):1885-1890.

Brennan, T. A., D. J. Rothman, L. Blank, D. Blumenthal, S. C. Chimonas, J. J. Cohen, J. Goldman, J. P. Kassirer, H. Kimball, J. Naughton, and N. Smelser. 2006. Health industry practices that create conflicts of interest: A policy proposal for academic medical centers. *Journal of the American Medical Association* 295(4):429-433.

Brosky, J. A., and R. Scott. 2007. Professional competence in physical therapy. *Journal of Allied Health* 36(2):113-118.

Coogle, L. 2008. *Perspectives on continuing education from providers and funders.* Presentation to the Committee on Planning a Continuing Health Care Professional Education Institute, December 11. Washington, DC: North American Association of Medical Education and Communication Companies.

Cooke, M., D. M. Irby, W. Sullivan, and K. M. Ludmerer. 2006. American medical education 100 years after the Flexner report. *New England Journal of Medicine* 355(13):1339-1344.

Davis, D., M. Evans, A. Jadad, L. Perrier, D. Rath, D. Ryan, G. Sibbald, S. Straus, S. Rappolt, M. Wowk, and M. Zwarenstein. 2003. The case for knowledge translation: Shortening the journey from evidence to effect. *British Medical Journal* 327(7405):33-35.

DeAngelis, C. D., and P. B. Fontanarosa. 2008. Impugning the integrity of medical science: The adverse effects of industry influence. *Journal of the American Medical Association* 299(15):1833-1835.

Grossman, J. 1998. Continuing competence in the health professions. *American Journal of Occupational Therapy* 52(9):709-715.

IOM (Institute of Medicine). 2009. *Conflict of interest in medical research, education, and practice.* Washington, DC: The National Academies Press.

Mazmanian, P. E. 2009. Commercial support of continuing medical education in the United States: The politics of doubt, the value of studies. *Journal of Continuing Education in the Health Professions* 29(2):81-83.

Mazmanian, P. E., D. E. Moore, R. M. Mansfield, and M. P. Neal. 1979. Perspectives on mandatory continuing medical education. *Southern Medical Journal* 72(4):378-380.

McCartney, M. 2004. The giving game: Do the freebies that doctors get from drugs companies affect the treatment they pick for patients? *Guardian* (May 25):10.

Michigan State Medical Society Committee on CME Accreditation. 2009. *Policy & procedure manual (a guide to the accreditation process).* East Lansing, MI: Michigan State Medical Society.

Miller, S. H., J. N. Thompson, P. E. Mazmanian, A. Aparicio, D. Davis, B. Spivey, and N. Kahn. 2008. Continuing medical education, professional development, and requirements for medical licensure: A white paper of the conjoint committee on continuing medical education. *Journal of Continuing Education in the Health Professions* 28(2):95-98.

NASW (National Association of Social Workers). 2003. *NASW standards for continuing professional education.* http://www.socialworkers.org/practice/standards/NASWContinuingEdStandards.pdf (accessed July 15, 2009).

Peck, C., M. McCall, B. McLaren, and T. Rotem. 2000. Continuing medical education and continuing professional development: International comparisons. *British Medical Journal* 320:432-435.

Peterson, E. D., K. M. Overstreet, J. N. Parochka, and M. R. Lemon. 2008. Medical education and communication companies in CME: An updated profile. *Journal of Continuing Education in the Health Professions* 24(8):205-219.

PhRMA (Pharmaceutical Research and Manufacturers of America). 2008. *Code on interactions with healthcare professionals.* Washington, DC: PhRMA.

Podolsky, S. H., and J. A. Greene. 2008. A historical perspective of pharmaceutical promotion and physician education. *Journal of the American Medical Association* 300(7):831-833.

Relman, A. S. 2001. Separating continuing medical education from pharmaceutical marketing. *Journal of the American Medical Association* 285(15):2009-2012.

Saxton, M. 2009. A view from industry: The foundations of future commercial support and a call for action. *Journal of Continuing Education in the Health Professions* 29(1):71-75.

Smith, J. L., R. M. Cervero, and T. Valentine. 2006. Impact of commercial support on continuing pharmacy education. *Journal of Continuing Education in the Health Professions* 26(4):302-312.

Steinbrook, R. 2005. Commercial support and continuing medical education. *New England Journal of Medicine* 352(6):534-535.

———. 2008. Financial support of continuing medical education. *Journal of the American Medical Association* 299(9):1060-1062.

United States Senate Committee on Finance. 2007. *Committee staff report to the chairman and ranking member: Use of educational grants by pharmaceutical manufacturers.* Washington, DC: U.S. Government Printing Office.

4

Moving Toward a Continuing Professional Development System

In its current state, continuing education (CE) does not help prepare health professionals to provide care that is of consistently high quality and improves patient outcomes. As detailed in the previous chapters, CE faces many problems, including:

- **The science underpinning CE for health professionals is fragmented and underdeveloped.** The lack of a strong science base makes it difficult if not impossible for health professionals to identify educational programs best suited to their needs, and the fragmentation of responsibility for research inhibits the establishment of a cohesive research agenda that can identify what works to best support continued learning.
- **The role and value of CE are not uniformly understood.** Health professionals who view CE merely as a mechanism for meeting regulatory requirements are missing the opportunity to attain goals of continued learning for improved practice. Regulators and the public also need to understand CE as a tool for improved practice.
- **There is concern about how CE is financed.** Of particular controversy is the role of funding from pharmaceutical and medical device companies and the possibility that such funding inherently creates conflicts of interest. Yet the present system has not identified alternative sources to replace dependence on industry financing.

- **In many cases, there is no relationship among the key regulatory components of state licensure, certification, credentialing, and accreditation.** Current regulatory processes generally exist as separate systems, leading to inconsistency, duplication, and confusion over what is needed to enhance learning. There is also little consensus about how effectively the regulatory processes are functioning.
- **Licensing requirements are inconsistent across states and professions.** The differences among state requirements do not have a scientific basis and thus reflect uncertainty about what amounts and types of CE are necessary, and in what contexts CE should be provided, for professionals to both maintain their competence and improve their practice.
- **CE lacks an established research agenda and is supported by a disrupted financing system,** making accreditation more difficult.
- **CE currently lacks a patient-based focus,** as quality and patient safety are not often well integrated into CE processes.
- **There is little recognition of the need for a multidisciplinary approach to CE.** Since health care requires collaboration among professionals, providing interprofessional education holds the most promise for better aligning learning with practice needs.

In sum, the current approach to CE has serious flaws. There are major gaps in research, regulation, and financing, and the components of CE are managed by different stakeholders operating in isolation. What is fundamentally needed is a coordinated vision of what an effective continuing professional development (CPD) system for health professions should entail—and the leadership to fulfill such a vision.

Many of the components of a comprehensive, broad-based CPD system are spelled out in previous chapters. This chapter will focus on ways to implement such a system.

ALTERNATIVES FOR REFORMING CONTINUING EDUCATION

In considering the establishment of an institute such as the one proposed in the committee's statement of task, the committee identified alternative means of improving health professions learning and evaluated whether the institute or another alternative was preferable. The committee focused on five alternatives:

1. Maintaining the status quo;
2. Developing a program within an existing government agency;
3. Forming a coalition of stakeholders;
4. Creating a new, private structure of professional societies; and
5. Developing a new, public-private structure.

The committee compared the ability of each alternative to achieve change in the following areas: research agenda, regulation, financing, conflict of interest, and interprofessional care (see Table 4-1). The committee also considered the long-term costs of the various alternatives.

Alternative 1: Maintaining the Status Quo

Maintaining the status quo would leave CE researchers, providers, funders, regulators, and other stakeholders to address problems facing CE on their own. Some important research topics, such as team-based learning and workplace learning, require a degree of collaboration that is difficult or impossible to achieve under the status quo. Research on the amounts and types of learning to best improve practitioner performance is also needed and currently is not identified as a responsibility of any one particular group or organization.

The fact that regulatory responsibilities for CE vary across jurisdictions and professions will impede necessary collaboration as well. Although some organizations are beginning to explore ways to work together, it remains clear that no central vision or force guides change and stakeholders have no incentive to move away from the status quo.

The inconsistency of financing across professions also limits the stability of CE in both the short and long terms. Under the status quo, financing does not support interprofessional learning, point of care learning, and other cross-cutting areas of learning. Moreover, although some policies have been developed recently, CE activities are not free from conflicted sources of funding. There is no mechanism to ensure that continued learning is free from conflicts of interest.

In addition, the status quo has limited capacity to promote widespread interprofessional learning opportunities. Some efforts exist in

TABLE 4-1 Overview of the Alternatives

| Alternative | Actors | Core Tasks | |
		Research agenda	Regulatory
Status quo	Current stakeholders	• No coordinated research agenda • Funding from potentially conflicted sources	• No central force to call for regulatory changes
Program within existing government agency	AHRQ	• Could provide focused investment in CE research and demonstration projects • Would promote close ties to QI	• Regulation not currently within its authority • Sensitivity about unilateral federal action to change state and professional roles
	HRSA	• Could invest in research and demonstration projects • Would promote close ties to research across education continuum	• Regulation not currently within its authority • Sensitivity about unilateral federal action to change state and professional roles
Coalition	Current stakeholders and other quality-focused organizations (e.g., NQF)	• No central convener • Could raise money to fund specific research areas • Could provide greater emphasis on QI	• Could develop voluntary regulatory standards

Financing	Conflict of interest	Interprofessional care
• No dedicated funding sources • 58 percent of funding for CE in medicine from pharmaceutical and medical device companies	• Some actions to reduce COI	• No incentives to promote team-based interprofessional care
• Would require change in mission to incorporate other sources of funding for CE • Historically unstable funding	• Lacks authority to make widespread impact on COI	• Could promote team-based interprofessional care
• Would require change in mission to incorporate other sources of funding for CE	• Lacks authority to make widespread impact on COI	• Addresses interprofessional education through Titles VII and VIII, but inconsistently
• Could result in more consistent funding • Could develop self-enforced financing regulations	• Could develop self-enforced COI guidelines	• Could promote interprofessional learning, but currently no strong research capacity to do so

continued

TABLE 4-1 Continued

| Alternative | Actors | Core Tasks | |
		Research agenda	Regulatory
New structure (private)	Societies of all health professions	• Professional societies fund own research, although somewhat limited • Could yield more profession-specific research	• Could directly influence certification and accreditation • Could work with others to enhance credentialing and licensure
New structure (public/private)	All deemed necessary to improve quality/patient safety	• Central agenda with coordinated priorities • Government/private foundations to fund	• Could coordinate stakeholder efforts to achieve better regulatory standards • Could conflict with efforts by states, professions, and/or employers

NOTE: AHRQ = Agency for Healthcare Research and Quality; CE = continuing education; COI = conflicts of interest; HRSA = Health Resources and Services Administration; NQF = National Quality Forum; QI = quality improvement.

the private sector through collaboration among some accrediting bodies. The public sector has also made investments through Title VII and Title VIII of the Public Health Service Act, administered by the Health Resources and Services Administration (HRSA), further discussed below. But none of these private or public activities has resulted in documented widespread improvements in health professional practice and patient outcomes, in part due to the inadequacies of the science, regulation, and financing of continuing education.

As to long-term costs, an important consideration that will help drive future CE efforts, there is no incentive under the status quo to reduce the costs or resources of CE activities and the overall CE system.

In view of the serious shortcomings of the status quo, the committee determined that it would be necessary to move toward some other alternative.

Financing	Conflict of interest	Interprofessional care
• Could result in more consistent funding • Could develop self-enforced financing regulations	• Could develop self-enforced COI guidelines	• Cross-cutting group could convene to set standards
• Could develop financing regulations and more consistent funding	• Could develop consensus COI guidelines	• Could promote interprofessional education

Alternative 2: Developing a Program Within an Existing Government Agency

The two federal agencies the committee considered most closely related to the issues of continuing education for health professionals are the Agency for Healthcare Research and Quality (AHRQ) and HRSA, both within the Department of Health and Human Services. A new program under one of these agencies could be given the authority to encourage collaboration, thereby setting a vision for all current stakeholders. Such a program could, to a degree, also work with current stakeholders to seek expert opinion and contract out some of its functions.

The Agency for Healthcare Research and Quality funds research to improve health care quality, safety, efficiency, and effectiveness. Its work includes research on evidence-based practice, development of guidelines, technology assessments, and comparative effectiveness—activities that overlap with continuing education. Placing the new program in the agency would explicitly link a research agenda for CPD to quality improvement. Translation from research to practice would also likely become a greater area of investigation, given AHRQ's past focus on knowledge translation. A program within AHRQ would be a good fit for development of a coordinated research agenda for CPD.

AHRQ's current mission does not include responsibility for coordination or regulation of CPD. It is also not within AHRQ's current charge to require adoption of strategies to reduce overall costs for private stakeholders. Assignment of these responsibilities to the agency would require action by Congress to establish both the authority and resources for this purpose. It is unlikely that Congress would create this authority in AHRQ, given the substantial vested interests in current arrangements by states, professional societies, and other stakeholders. Alternatively, AHRQ could collaborate or contract with current groups (e.g., Accreditation Council on Continuing Medical Education, National Association of Boards of Pharmacy) to develop a system that would allow it to be involved with regulatory and financing activities.

The Health Resources and Services Administration focuses on improving access to culturally competent, high quality health care. Among its activities, HRSA provides grants to reinforce the health care workforce. This includes providing some funds for continuing education and professional development made available through Title VII and Title VIII of the Public Health Service Act. Specific to continuing education, Title VII provides money for the Area Health Education Center program that, among other things, trains health professionals working in underserved populations and local communities and supports interprofessional education and training. Title VIII focuses on the nursing workforce and funds some continuing education through the Nurse Education, Practice, and Retention Grants program and the Comprehensive Geriatric Education Grants program.

HRSA's capacity to develop and administer a CPD research agenda is promising, given its focus on workforce and experience in postlicensure training through the previously described programs. Placing a CPD program in HRSA would foster greater linkages in research along the entire learning continuum, supporting the notion of lifelong learning. Its work on interprofessional health care also makes it a plausible candidate to guide a new CPD system.

However, HRSA does not presently have the authority to address regulation, financing, conflicts of interest, or long-term costs of a

CPD system. It could be involved in setting and administering a research agenda, but managing a full CPD system would require major changes to the mission of HRSA.

In either agency, a new program would benefit from having a system already in place to carry out a research agenda. The program would need to carefully set priorities and work with current stakeholders to minimize duplication of effort between the private and public sectors. Such a program would need strong leadership and careful planning to fully benefit from the expertise of the current system. Of particular concern are the preemption of the roles of states and professional associations and the need to greatly expand the agency's mission. The committee therefore concluded that the government-run alternative would not be able to address the range of problems in the current CE system.

Alternative 3: Forming a Coalition

The beginnings of this option already may be in place, as some CE stakeholders have joined together for specific professions (e.g., Conjoint Committee on Continuing Medical Education). Groups of this nature could be the basis for building a broader coalition, including organizations whose purposes are to improve health care quality and patient safety, such as the National Committee for Quality Assurance (NCQA) and the National Quality Forum (NQF). This voluntary coalition would extend the current group of stakeholders to include others able to contribute significantly to developing a comprehensive CPD system.

Formation of such a coalition would bring CPD more squarely in line with the goal of improving quality and patient safety. With respect to a research agenda, the coalition could raise money to fund specific research priorities and develop a coordinated agenda. Research monies would continue to be raised through private organizations and the government.

Regulation of CPD by a coalition of stakeholders could provide an opportunity for stakeholders to work together toward better regulatory standards. More harmonized regulations could be developed through the inherent collaborative work of a coalition. It could strengthen linkages among accreditation, certification, credentialing, and licensure systems within each profession and across health professions.

A coalition could also improve the CPD financing structure. The collaborative nature could result in more consistent funding and generate mechanisms for more focused funding. Identification of additional sources of financing could also occur due to the broader group of stakeholders.

Conflicts of interest could also be addressed by such a coalition. For instance, a subgroup could develop financing guidelines to promote conflict-free CPD activities and build on current efforts. However, in this strategy, conflict of interest guidelines would likely be self-enforced.

While a coalition would be interprofessional in nature, interprofessional education and development may not be actively supported. Clear goals toward the advancement of interprofessional learning would need to be delineated. Strong leadership would also need to be identified to successfully support such an agenda. Unless interprofessional, team-based learning is set as a high priority goal, it will not be achieved, because the current incentives for a coalition to support it are inadequate to foster widespread change.

Although long-term costs could be reduced in this alternative, it is not within a voluntary coalition's direct ability to reduce costs and resource use unless it is made a specific goal. Each stakeholder would have the option of supporting decreasing costs in the system, but no overarching source of accountability would exist.

A coalition has many positive attributes that would make it a reasonable option to develop and spearhead a CPD system, but it may take many years to develop because of the complexity of the status quo. There is no clear authority capable of pulling these groups together. There is also no precedent in this field to support the notion that all groups would agree on similar goals for a CPD system without such an authority. The lack of leadership and incentive for these groups to work with one another may dilute the focus of immediately developing a CPD system, leading to more of the same. Because the committee believes that advancing the system in an effective manner will require strong leadership, this alternative was not recommended.

Alternative 4: Creating a New, Private Structure

In this scenario, the new structure would be operated by professional societies and organizations across all health professions. The professions would collectively base decisions about the development of a CPD system on their expertise. Supporting the professions would be at the forefront of such a structure. It could collaborate with other stakeholders (e.g., employers, researchers, state boards, funders) to build the remaining infrastructure needed to support a CPD system.

A research agenda developed by this structure has the capacity to strengthen research on teams and interprofessional care. It would also foster strong ties between the research agenda and professionals' practice needs. However, a CPD research agenda developed in such a structure may become subject to the political agendas of each profession, instead of enhancing an interprofessional approach. Orienting a research agenda toward improving quality and patient safety in this alternative would be more difficult to achieve as compared to the coalition described in Alternative 3.

A private structure managed by professional societies would likely drive greater coordination and standardization in certification and accreditation, compared with the alternatives of the status quo and a government-operated program. It is also likely that this structure could collaborate with state boards and employers to align with the licensure and credentialing systems.

In a structure operated by professional societies, more consistent funding could be developed, and greater coordination among professions could address concerns about the currently varied financing mechanisms. Conflict of interest guidelines could also be set across the health professions. But without central leadership, these guidelines would be self-enforced without a source of accountability, leaving the integrity of the system in question.

Interprofessional care would need to be identified as a priority. Without agreement by all professions, each profession may indeed advocate for itself and not for shared learning environments and team-based care.

A private structure would not have the ability or authority to reduce the long-term costs of a CPD system. Stakeholders are all separated without an incentive to promote change.

The development of a structure operated by professional societies shares some of the same benefits of the coalition alternative, perhaps the most important being the ability to explicitly seek input of those representing health professionals. (However, the private structure would not engage as many other stakeholders as the coalition.) A private structure also would share some of the negative aspects of the coalition, such as lack of leadership to coordinate and align efforts. Without a source of authority to hold the structure accountable, it would be difficult to implement a culture of continued learning. Given the current state, the committee concludes that a private structure formed by the professional societies, like the coalition alternative, does not have an impetus to come together and make an impact in a timely manner.

Alternative 5: Developing a New, Public-Private Structure

All of the prior alternatives could lead to improvements in CE. But none strikes a good balance between a collaborative effort going forward and recognizing the role of professional societies and other stakeholders. The committee therefore concluded that a hybrid strategy that yields the benefits of the first four alternatives but is structured to avoid the negatives is needed to make timely progress toward a comprehensive, effective CPD system.

A new, public-private structure is just such a hybrid. The goal of such a structure would be to convene and work with the stakeholders, not preempt them. The presumed federal role in a public-private structure would be to convene relevant groups and develop a mechanism to hold them responsible for achieving an aligned set of goals toward creating an improved CPD system. A broad group of stakeholders—including states, the professions, employers of health professionals, and organizations that focus on quality and patient safety—would collectively develop and work toward improving quality and patient safety, while building on their collective expertise to create a collaborative culture of CPD.

The structure would have the capacity to build a comprehensive research agenda and set priorities across all health professions. Similar to the coalition and private structure alternatives, it would have more consistent sources of research funding through a pooled approach. The number of activities sponsored by conflicted sources could also be greatly reduced upon broad adoption of conflict of interest policies.

In a public-private structure, current bodies in charge of licensure, certification, credentialing, and accreditation would continue in their roles but would also work together to develop better regulatory standards based on research findings. The goal of such a structure would be to convene and work with the stakeholders, not preempt them. For example, a model could be implemented that would enable states to provide input to the development of regulatory standards, but each state would retain authority to modify its laws, make any changes to its own regulatory processes, and find the resources needed to institute changes. A process could be established analogous to the National Association of Insurance Commissioners, which develops model laws that are then passed to the states to either adopt in their entirety or modify to meet the needs of the local circumstances. These model laws have served to encourage the collaboration of states on issues surrounding the insurance commissioners' roles through committees and task forces. Further, organizations that represent the state boards, such as the Federation of State Medical Boards and its equivalent bodies, would participate with other regulatory bodies in the development of widely agreed upon standards and goals for CPD.

A somewhat analogous organization is the National Quality Forum, a not-for-profit membership organization that convenes stakeholders to endorse measures of health care quality. The NQF was developed by the 1998 President's Commission on Consumer Protection and Quality in the Health Care Industry. The commission recognized the need to develop standards for measuring health care quality and performance because of the promulgation of numerous highly varied sets of measures, resulting in unreliable data on which to base decisions. The NQF was established with private funding matched by the Department of Health and Human Services to oversee development of measures of health care quality, data collection, and reporting. A structure of councils is used to obtain input from its member stakeholders.

This alternative is more complex than the others and would therefore be more complicated to implement. Active participation and acceptance by a wide range of stakeholders would be needed to identify and implement changes. Developing a public-private structure would likely be resource-intensive, although a more coordinated CPD system would more efficiently and effectively manage resource utilization in the long term, resulting in a higher-value system compared to a system without such leadership.

The committee concludes that with strong leadership, a new public-private partnership is the best alternative to effect change. The committee therefore calls on the federal government to work with current stakeholders and act as the initial convener to stimulate change toward the development of a public-private central body tasked with integrating the key components of CPD. The Secretary of the Department of Health and Human Services should take the lead, but also should coordinate with directors of other government bodies such as the Department of Veterans Affairs and the Department of Education.

Recommendation 1: The Secretary of the Department of Health and Human Services should, as soon as practical, commission a planning committee to develop a public-private institute for continuing health professional development. The resulting institute should coordinate and guide efforts to align approaches in the areas of:
(a) Content and knowledge of CPD among health professions,

(b) **Regulation across states and national CPD providers,**
(c) **Financing of CPD for the purpose of improving professional performance and patient outcomes, and**
(d) **Development and strengthening of a scientific basis for the practice of CPD.**

The institute, which the IOM committee has called the Continuing Professional Development Institute (CPDI), should be designed as a neutral body that promotes and catalyzes collaboration. With the benefit of stakeholder input, dedicated resources, and sufficient time in which to plan and develop a CPDI, a planning committee should be commissioned as soon as determined by the Secretary.

CONCLUSION

Continuing education is deeply embedded in both the public and private sectors. Of the alternatives the committee considered, only the hybrid public-private structure recognized the tensions and relationships that exist among stakeholders. The committee has no illusion that the CPDI is a perfect option or that generating the continuing financial commitment from the government or private sector stakeholders will be an easy task. But the committee believes that mounting a carefully planned, strong effort to improve continuing professional development across health professions is worth the effort and will result in better and safer care for patients.

5

Envisioning a Better System of Continuing Professional Development

T he Institute of Medicine's (IOM's) report *Health Professions Education: A Bridge to Quality* (2003) called for improving the health care workforce and affirmed the quintessential value of education and training in advancing this mission. The report recommended a set of five competencies that all health professionals should possess. Ensuring that health professionals attain and maintain these competencies should be at the heart of a new continuing professional development (CPD) system, which would hold as its ultimate aim improving patient outcomes and protecting patient safety. As outlined briefly in previous chapters, an effective CPD system should ensure that health professionals are prepared to:

1. *Provide patient-centered care.* At its core, a CPD system will embody an ethical commitment to ensuring health and patient safety. CPD holds the promise of equipping clinicians with powerful tools to better communicate with patients, while strengthening their ability to advocate for disease prevention and wellness. CPD will enable clinicians to more easily keep pace with the evolving evidence base relating to their patients' diverse values, preferences, backgrounds, and well-being.
2. *Work in interprofessional teams.* Team-based learning and training will be central to promote coordination and collaboration across health professions, helping them to learn with, from,

and about one another. Effective coordination and use of interprofessional teams of practitioners in the care setting requires practice and the development of a collaborative skill set that is not routinely taught at other levels of health professions education. Imparting such proficiencies should be a key feature of a CPD system.

3. *Employ evidence-based practice.* New knowledge generated by health research is a potent driver of CPD, providing rich sources of information in learning. Advances in health care can be made when research identifies and fills knowledge gaps. Clinical outcomes data for individual, team, and institutional assessment can identify the successes and areas of inadequacies of current practice, lay the groundwork for improvement, and continuously guide the evolution of a strengthened system of care.

4. *Apply quality improvement.* All professionals in health care should aim for continuous improvement of their performance to deliver the best patient care. CPD should model principles of quality improvement by continuously evaluating the quality of structure, processes, and outcomes of CPD activities. The CPD system will benefit when its providers and researchers collaborate with other professionals in the quality improvement community; efficiencies gained from such collaborations could yield important benefits to patients. For example, grounding the quality improvement efforts of health professionals into proven educational techniques will provide systems-based feedback to planners, policy makers, and participating health professionals. Through this collaboration, CPD can serve as a precise tool in the learning health care system, supporting provision of care toward the six quality aims.

5. *Use health informatics.* Modern health information technologies provide an unprecedented opportunity for capturing and rapidly analyzing real-time data at the point of care to help clinicians manage data, improve safety, make informed clinical decisions, and access information or community resources. The field of health informatics encompasses e-learning, electronic data collection, collation and analysis, electronic decision support, and information management from individuals to populations to illuminate best practices in health service delivery. The CPD system will enlist these resources to advance learning and quality care.

VISION FOR A SYSTEM OF
CONTINUING PROFESSIONAL DEVELOPMENT

An effective continuing professional development system would offer significant improvement over today's fragmented approach to continuing education. Whereas the current funding of CE by commercial groups may hold inherent conflicts of interest that shift the focus away from improving health professionals' performance, a CPD system would promote patient-centered care. Moreover, a CPD system would help obviate some of CE's current fragmentation by driving coordination of activities and fostering interprofessional teams. A CPD system would be thoroughly evidence-based in its delivery, innovation, and research, representing a marked change from the current disconnect between CE theory, research, and practice that have resulted in few evidence-based activities to support health professionals' competence and patient outcomes. A CPD system would help clinicians achieve quality improvement, while peer-reviewed studies of CE can claim to support only minimum levels of competence and have infrequently proven effective for improving the quality of care. Although CE has minimally used health information technologies in training and education, a comprehensive CPD system would foster development and dissemination of technology-based approaches.

The structure of the CPD system needs to support the system's goals and deliver systematic and timely information to health professionals based on their learning needs and the challenges they encounter in clinical practice. First, CPD research must be driven by learning theory inclusive of insights and advances from the social, biological, and health sciences. Second, funding for CPD should be guided by sound economic principles and should set a goal of improving patient outcomes, not promoting a particular product or service. Third, implementing an effective CPD system will require mobilizing the CPD enterprise to promote a culture of learning for patient care. Fourth, the CPD system must be accountable and transparent to the public.

In a comprehensive CPD system, individual health practitioners would be committed to and take control over their own professional development and learning. Achieving this will require making the system learner-driven and more responsive to learners' requirements and flexible enough to adapt to the learning opportunities that present with the ever-changing needs of patients.

CPD needs to facilitate health professionals' learning beyond the classroom and professional conferences. It must be an ongoing process that occurs at the point of care, in conversations with colleagues, and in the many other ways that clinicians resolve daily problems of patient care. A high-performing system would recognize that health professions education is not limited to formal educational activities and must integrate with the learning that health professionals internalize in their everyday practice.

CPD also must be tailored to the various stages of a health professional's career. The learning needs and opportunities of novice health practitioners should be differentiated from those of intermediate or expert practitioners. These stages of expertise, defined by topics and experience, carry important implications for educational design. These processes are much more complex than simply knowing or not knowing. On a finer scale, knowledge of any clinical skill can be broken down into four progressive stages:

1. Declarative knowledge: the learner gains the awareness to identify a problem or to know what should be done;
2. Procedural knowledge: the learner not only understands that there is a problem to solve but also gains knowledge of how to go about solving it;
3. Competence: the learner advances to a stage where he can demonstrate or show how a problem is to be solved; and
4. Performance: the learner identifies the problem, knows how to address it, demonstrates the needed skill, and solves the problem in practice—the learner does what he has learned.

These stages of skill acquisition can serve as a useful framework for the assessment of clinical skill development (see Figure 5-1) (Moore et al., 2009).

As a fundamental requirement, all health professionals should understand the value of CPD and incorporate CPD into their careers. The importance of CPD should be infused as individuals enter their health professional training and should be reinforced and sustained throughout their careers. The tenets of CPD should therefore be anchored by lifelong learning. Understanding the importance of CPD through prelicensure training helps to firmly secure this pursuit as a lifelong professional commitment and a vitally important educational practice of responsible health professionals.

The CPD system should address clinicians' learning needs at the point of care where practice-based inquiry and the learning needs of clinicians originate, and CPD methods should provide the skills or tools required to meet those needs. The system needs to further efforts to develop valid and reliable measures for assessing the progress of learners, the associated health care outcomes of patients, and

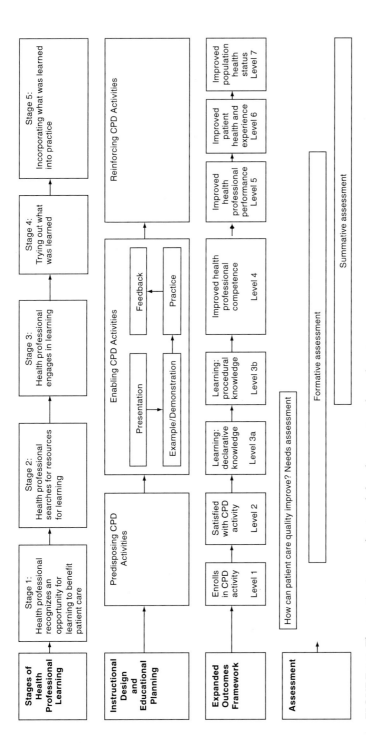

FIGURE 5-1 The continuing professional development cycle and system.
SOURCE: Adapted from Moore et al., 2009.

the value of the CPD system in improving health care. Figure 5-1 recognizes that health professionals' learning needs are not all alike and that specific skills are necessary to meet specific needs. Different instructional design and educational plans will be required, depending on the given learning opportunity and stage of learning. Targeted learning methods can be used to teach a particular skill, from predisposing activities, to enabling activities, to reinforcing activities. As discussed in Chapter 2, appropriate outcomes, such as improvement in a health professional's learning and/or behavior change, exist along a spectrum of outcomes levels. Proper use of targeted tools will lead to effective CPD, but not all learning activities are appropriate to advance all types of skills and to achieve all varieties of outcomes in all contexts. Resultant outcomes must be assessed to determine their value in specific contexts to the individual practitioner's learning or performance, patient health, and population health.

After the formative assessment of the value of CPD outcomes, a summative needs assessment brings the CPD cycle back to where it began, with the identification of a new set of practice-based learning needs to be addressed through another round of tailored CPD (see Box 5-1 for an example). A CPD system based on this cycle will meet the needs of individual health professionals and the health care system to improve quality and patient safety.

> **Recommendation 2: To achieve the new vision of a continuing professional development system, the planning committee should design an institute that:**
> (a) Creates a new scientific foundation for CPD to enhance health professionals' ability to provide better care;
> (b) Develops, collects, analyzes, and disseminates metrics, including process and outcome measures unique to CPD;
> (c) Encourages development and use of health information technology and emerging electronic health databases as a means to provide feedback on professionals' and health system performance;
> (d) Encourages development and sharing of improvement tools (e.g., learning portfolios, assessment resources) and theories of knowledge and practice (e.g., peer review systems for live documentation, such as wikis) across professions;
> (e) Fosters interprofessional collaboration to create and evaluate CPD programs and processes; and

---

BOX 5-1
CPD: One Surgeon's Performance and Value

A well-respected general surgeon at a community hospital subscribes to her profession's major journal and reads the articles thoroughly to keep up with advances in the field. She is particularly impressed with the results of one study of a new laparoscopic procedure showing significantly shortened hospital length of stay compared to open surgery. Reading the study carefully, she notes that it was performed at a major academic medical center whose staff had had many months of experience performing the procedure prior to the study. She would like to provide the same benefit to her patients that was found in the study, but recognizes that she and her staff are inexperienced with the new laparoscopic procedure and might do harm to patients while learning.

This surgeon identified a specific learning need (practice of the laparoscopic procedure) for a patient-centered care goal, requiring a tailored continuing professional development (CPD) activity to achieve the needed training. At this point, it is important to recognize that the surgeon already had completed at least one CPD cycle related to the procedure: she learned of the procedure by reading her professional journal, assessed the value of this knowledge in her individual practice setting, and performed a needs assessment to identify the need for greater practice with the procedure before actually performing it. In this case, a surgical simulator CPD activity would allow needed practice of the laparoscopic technique by the surgeon and her team, avoid harm to patients that might accrue if the surgeon had simply attended lectures before attempting the procedure, and benefit the community hospital's patients through a shorter hospital length of stay.

(f) **Improves the value and cost-effectiveness of CPD delivery and considering ways to relate the outputs of CPD to the quality and safety of the health care system.**

STEPS TO ENHANCE CONTINUING PROFESSIONAL DEVELOPMENT

The steps needed to support this vision include developing a new scientific foundation of CPD, developing new measures to assess CPD and its impact, developing and implementing health information technologies, identifying effective education improvement tools, enhancing interprofessional collaboration, and generating the "value proposition" for CPD that fully captures the value of CPD in improving health care quality and patient safety.

Developing a New Scientific Foundation for CPD

CE research is fragmented, may overlook insights from educational theory, and typically focuses too narrowly on professional learning in nonclinical contexts. CE research methods incorporate both qualitative and quantitative research designs. Research topics include the identification of theoretical constructs of change and learning and the measurement of improved patient outcomes associated with planned educational interventions. The construct of CPD refers to the body of concepts, variables, and theories that underlie the field. However, the current evidence inadequately answers questions regarding the effectiveness of learning activities and does not provide clear guidance for investing in CPD. A review of the research agenda and improvements in research will be critical to the success of the CPD system. Greater emphasis must be placed on integrating CPD research efforts that already exist, as well as on developing further research capabilities to create a new construct for CPD. Stronger research on theory, methods, and outcomes related to CPD will be the foundation for progress. This construct ought to improve health outcomes by effectively translating knowledge to support a continuous loop of research to inform practice and practice to inform research.

To facilitate understanding and evaluation of CPD techniques, CPD researchers need to adopt a common framework, whether focused on the educational theory supporting CPD or its clinical application. This framework should incorporate insights regarding CPD that have been gleaned from diverse disciplines, including adult education, psychology, sociology, health informatics, and organizational change. It also should integrate and harmonize the terminology and taxonomy used to describe CE methods in the health professions literature, employed by accreditors, and used by the various health professions. This step would result in a much-needed common language to facilitate communication and mutual collaboration toward building a new and shared culture of CPD.

A high-performing CPD system requires a stronger scientific foundation of CPD and includes a comprehensive research agenda to systematically identify gaps in evidence at the patient, practitioner, organizational, and societal levels. Once identified, these gaps should be pursued as opportunities and addressed through improvements in health professionals' knowledge, skills, and attitudes. Coordination of efforts would be emphasized to streamline the generation and dissemination of innovations and reduce unwitting duplication of research efforts.

Developing New Measures to Assess CPD and Its Impact

A measurement system needs to be established to assess CPD and its impact on health professionals' performance, which would provide needed guidance for investing in CPD. Measures should facilitate the identification and teaching of skills required to meet educational needs, and alignment of good learning and good health care. The measurement of CPD should allow for straightforward assessment at the higher levels of outcomes (Moore et al., 2009). Data from this measurement system should serve to enhance evidence-based CPD and the existing quality measurement enterprise, bridging the two fields, promoting their collaboration, and helping to ensure cross-disciplinary communication.

Developing standardized measures would represent an important step toward developing robust assessment of CPD, and an interprofessional approach to measure development will be important. Because CPD exists at the unique intersection of fields including health care, education, and the social sciences, metrics that match the unique nature of CPD will need to be developed. In a comprehensive CPD system, measures for evaluation of impact and value would be collected. Studies of costs, effects, and benefits of CPD would accelerate and more fully integrate CPD with systematic efforts involving quality improvement and patient safety. Organizations such as the National Quality Forum, the Agency for Healthcare Research and Quality, the National Committee for Quality Assurance, and the Institute for Healthcare Improvement, which have developed an infrastructure to set priorities, create and endorse performance measures, and publicly report data to improve care quality, would benefit from the additional resource of CPD in helping to assure the application and measurement of innovation in clinical practice.

Developing and Implementing Health Information Technologies

Over the past decade, modern health information technology has created innovative ways to support CPD. Computers, mobile computing devices (e.g., personal digital assistants, smart phones), computer networks linked through the Internet, and simulators have demonstrated their utility to help individuals and groups in their CPD. These tools can provide powerful knowledge acquisition opportunities, realistic simulations of case scenarios, unprecedented computer modeling and gaming for individual and team skills training, and timely data collection for audit and reflection. Further, decision support software accessible through computer or mobile technologies and social networking environments can amply support

---

BOX 5-2
Examples of Technology-Enabled CPD

Current examples of technology-enabled continuing professional development (CPD) approaches and the gradual accumulation of evidence to support their effectiveness include the following:

- *e-Learning courses or short learning points*: Well-designed e-learning courses can be as good as or better than traditional learning methods for individual practitioners, as measured by learner satisfaction, knowledge retention, and even skills acquisition (Cook et al., 2008; Fordis et al., 2005). The positive learning effects of e-learning are attributed to several reasons, including learner-dictated pacing of the activity to tailor to different individuals' speed of knowledge acquisition, ability to replay parts or all of the learning session without affecting the quality or authenticity of the educational experience, and nonlinear structure of the learning materials to allow learners to take their own approaches to content exploration. Additional advantages of e-learning include accessibility to learning unrestricted by time of day and geographic location of the learners, as well as the multimedia nature for capturing educational materials.
- *Electronic data collection and analysis*: Electronic data collection can be used to help clinicians analyze their practice patterns to identify gaps in performance that must be filled through CPD. Handheld electronic devices will allow clinicians to immediately learn about clinical problems, taking advantage of the teachable moment. Data systems to help clinicians track their own progress through CPD cycles already exist, representing promising ways to make high quality CPD accessible to all.
- *Simulation*: Technology-enabled simulation can include but is not limited to Internet-based case scenarios to unfold a journey of a

---

tailored, just-in-time information and knowledge exchange opportunities for unstructured learning or tacit knowledge acquisition.

With the emerging technology-enabled CPD initiatives described in Box 5-2 and other initiatives, a new world of learning can be developed and integrated into learning environments for knowledge capture, dissemination, transmission, and reflection. These approaches and those using other emerging technologies, such as smart phones or social networking approaches, ought to be rigorously studied to validate their efficacy in supporting learning and, if found effective, integrated into mainstream CPD.

patient case with embedded learning points, programmable high fidelity mannequins for realistic simulation of an actual patient, virtual reality to simulate patient procedures, or computer modeling of a population of patients in cases of infectious disease management or hospital patient flow management scenarios. All of these simulations share the same CPD advantage of preserving the authenticity and reproducibility of the learning experiences to standardize administration and learning points.

- *Longitudinal data*: Population data such as those collected by electronic health records (about a patient longitudinally from different sources such as hospitals or clinics over time) or personal health records (longitudinal electronic records that patients assemble themselves, consisting of data from their health professionals and their own interpretations) provide mechanisms through which health professionals can access the health outcomes of patients they have treated and the resultant effects. For example, physicians can determine how many of their diabetic patients consistently measure hemoglobin A1c, a standard of care. Over time, these data will help reflect not only how often they follow guidelines, but also how much they improve over time.
- *e-Mentoring*: Mentoring at the point of care, such as telemedicine consultations when the patients receive care while the clinician learns from the consultant, can be used to enhance learning.
- *Social networking*: Social networking sites such as Twitter and Facebook provide the opportunity for health professionals to communicate, collaborate, and share ideas with each other and the public in unparalleled ways—with additional possibilities yet unknown. These sites have the capacity to reach much larger audiences, are relatively convenient to use, and can have the potential to create new communities of learning. The promise of social networking tools cannot be ignored and should be embraced.

Identifying Effective Education Improvement Tools

Research has already made significant progress in identifying effective education methods. The attributes and principles of effective CE interventions noted in Chapter 2 include needs assessments to guide CPD providers and learners, interactivity, continuous integrated feedback, and the use of multiple learning methods. These attributes and principles are well known (Davis et al., 1999, 2006; Marinopoulos et al., 2007; Ratanawongsa et al., 2008), but little effort has been made to systematically translate them into practice so they can be broadly applied to CPD learning activities. Research on CPD needs to build on this existing knowledge base for effective learning and should encourage the application of such research to improve the effectiveness of CPD methods.

A better system would identify effective learning activities based on standardized, transparent pilot testing and evaluation of resultant learning, performance improvement, and patient outcomes. Once promising CPD activities are shown to be effective, implementation mechanisms need to be developed and robust measures should be employed to determine their impact on patients and professionals.

The CPD system will seek to promote innovative learning strategies at the health professional, organizational, and systems levels. Innovation needs to be rewarded through research that pilots and disseminates promising new methods and employs standardized monitoring of impact. Lifelong learning, practice-based learning, workplace learning, and learning portfolios are examples of innovations in CPD that have significant promise for advancing the science of performance improvement based on existing evidence.

- *Lifelong learning* is a necessary practice for any health professional, because of the rapidly advancing state of knowledge in all health care fields. There may be no more central skill for CPD than the ability to identify questions to be addressed in one's practice, independently muster resources to address those problems, and reassess one's learning needs as a matter of common practice. These skills typify the lifelong learner.
- *Practice-based learning* is a term applied to any learning activity whose material for study and improvement is the practitioner's workplace or panel of patients. Practice-based learning ensures that the skills and knowledge gained by professional learners are relevant to the patients they care for and their problems. As a result, practice-based learning has a higher probability of positively impacting those same patients.
- *Workplace learning* emerges in a just-in-time fashion as part of everyday work activities. Workplace learning may be useful in preventing errors, supporting a culture of reflection on and in action, and encouraging sustained learning environments.
- *Learning portfolios* are based on the adult learning principle of analysis of and reflection on experience. They enable practicing health professionals to document, formally assess, and learn from their clinical and educational experiences. Learning portfolios can be either web-based or exist in hard copy. As interactive professional development tools, some portfolios have built in milestones of accomplishment that can inform patients, the public, and regulators of the experiences

of a professional. Learning portfolios have been effectively used in a variety of learning environments (e.g., visual arts students, K-12 and college education). Specific to health care, learning portfolios were first adopted by nurses and midwives and have now spread to other health professions, especially in the United Kingdom, and they have been adopted in the United States by the Accreditation Council for Graduate Medical Education in the case of medical residents. They offer much promise to support lifelong learning for all health professionals.

Enhancing Interprofessional Collaboration

Collaboration among professions is necessary for the provision of optimal health care in modern health care settings (see Box 5-3). Interprofessional education through CPD can be the transformative force to promote and inspire seamless collaboration, help diffuse advances across fields, and optimize the way professionals operate, both individually and jointly. Interprofessional education is defined as "any type of educational training, teaching, or learning session in which two or more health and social care professions are learning interactively" (Reeves et al., 2009). Interprofessional education therefore not only educates clinicians from multiple professions together but also fosters the development of a culture that promotes interprofessional, team-based care for improved health care quality and patient safety. This culture shift cannot occur in isolation in the CPD community, but it will be critical throughout the trajectory of health professionals' lifelong learning.

CPD is an ideal forum through which collaboration can promote team-based care, and greater inclusion can spark synergistic advances among professionals' knowledge. At no other stage of health professionals' training are they as exposed to, dependent on, and accountable to members of the health care team from professions other than their own. The greater amount of interaction and interdependence with other professions makes CPD a logical stage at which to foreground interprofessional collaboration and education. CPD methods can reduce barriers between professional silos, allowing interprofessional collaboration to carry over into practice.

Generating the Value Proposition for CPD

Demonstrating the value or business case for CPD is largely unexplored at present; its value will be in improving health care

BOX 5-3
Interprofessional Team-Based Learning and Care

The stroke team at Saybrook Hospital took part in a CPD training initiative in care coordination that included group process analysis and quality improvement workplace learning discussions.

The primary team consisted of the neurology service, intensivists, nursing personnel, radiology, ICU (intensive care unit) pharmacists, and respiratory therapy. The team studied the case of a stroke patient, upon presentation to the emergency room (ER) and transfer to the ICU. On assessment, the team discovered underlying, poorly controlled hypertension that contributed to the stroke, and the cardiology service was added to the team. In following this case over a prolonged hospital stay, roles of multiple team members were identified: the ICU team of physicians, respiratory therapists managing the patient's mechanical ventilation, neurology service, nursing staff, physical and occupational therapists performing serial functional assessments, a nutritionist approving a low-salt diet to address the underlying hypertension, and the cardiology team ordering new medication to control the patient's blood pressure. The team discussed how to share the care plan and other pertinent data needed to assess and recommend therapies and patient education.

As the case progressed to discharge, blood pressure medication was titrated to the optimal dose, dietary changes were established, and referrals made for follow-up disease management services and a course of physical therapy. Upon recognizing that the only physical therapy facility accepting the patient's health insurance was 20 miles from the patient's home, the team strategized ways to facilitate care delivery and effectively transition to the patient's primary care team.

Soon after completing the CPD exercise, a patient with a major stroke was admitted through the ER to the ICU. Due to the lessons learned through CPD, the inpatient team implemented the identified strategies to enhance collaboration and deliver high quality care. The primary care doctor informed the inpatient team that the patient's respiratory condition had been exacerbated by similar blood pressure medications in the past, and the cardiology team found an alternate blood pressure regimen. The primary care physician also informed the inpatient team that the patient did not have access to transportation to the physical therapy facility, prompting the inpatient physical therapist to arrange for care through a clinical trial at a nearby academic stroke rehabilitation center. The outpatient nutritionist was able to use the hospital nutritionist's initial assessment and make needed adjustments rather than starting from scratch.

These adjustments improved the quality of the care that this hypothetical patient received, as the result of team-based training through CPD.

quality and patient safety. The value proposition for CE can be derived through its profit generation for academic centers, professional societies, industry, and the public. The value of CPD to the patient paying for care and to the health practitioner must also be considered, as well as the value to the health care system as a whole. Metrics to determine the value of CPD need to be developed, including clear methods of determining the impacts of CPD on the quality and cost of care. Ultimately, arriving at the value proposition for CPD will be essential to understanding the best ways to invest CPD resources.

COLLABORATION WITH STAKEHOLDERS FOR HEALTH CARE QUALITY

Both interprofessional and intraprofessional collaboration are necessary for a high performing CPD system. To maximize the quality of learning, organizations and groups driving continuing education need to work in synergy to develop a more effective and efficient system (see Box 5-4 for an example in medicine). Such programs ought to be organized within each health profession, coordinated with those of other health professions, and ultimately work in partnership with other health care organizations. The committee believes collaboratives are important to the functions of a CPD system and need to work with other organizations that have the funding and authority to pull the various stakeholders together from all relevant health professions.

A culture of learning to support quality will span both the CPD system and the quality improvement community. To benefit CPD, those in quality improvement should use the infrastructure already in place for data collection and reporting mechanisms. This relationship is logical: CPD is a major component of specialty certification, licensure, and credentialing for privileges and includes educational systems that are important for the dissemination of clinical innova tions and knowledge derived from quality improvement and quality improvement research. The drive for competence and continuous improvement of service is integral to professionalism and the lifelong pursuit of knowledge. The benefits that each domain contributes to the other could be mutually reinforcing and exponentially accrued.

Others involved in CPD, including funders, providers, and regulators, share the common aims of optimizing health professional knowledge and patient health outcomes. A highly collaborative approach among these groups would likely drive more effi-

---

BOX 5-4
Example of a Collaborative on
Continuing Medical Education (CME)

The Conjoint Committee on Continuing Medical Education (Conjoint Committee) has advocated for reform of continuing medical education, recommending that leaders of organized medicine address accreditation, certification, credentialing, licensure, and funding of CME (Spivey, 2005). The Conjoint Committee recently proposed that each medical specialty and subspecialty should develop competency-based curricula to support member learning, self-assessment, and continuing competence (Jackson et al., 2007) and that state medical boards should require valid and reliable assessment of physicians' learning needs (Miller et al., 2008). Most recently, the Conjoint Committee recommended that research in continuing medical education should be raised to a national priority (Miller et al., 2008). Member organizations include the following:

Accreditation Council for Continuing Medical Education
Alliance for Continuing Medical Education
American Academy of Family Physicians
American Board of Medical Specialties
American Hospital Association
American Medical Association
American Osteopathic Association
Association for Hospital Medical Education
Association of American Medical Colleges
Council of Medical Specialty Societies
Federation of State Medical Boards
Society for Academic Continuing Medical Education

Four other member groups are participants in the Conjoint Committee but are not full voting members: Accreditation Council for Graduate Medical Education, *Journal of Continuing Education in the Health Professions*, National Board of Medical Examiners, and The Joint Commission.

---

cient resource allocation and increase the value of available CPD activities.

Recommendation 3: The planning committee should design the Continuing Professional Development Institute to work with other entities whose purpose is to improve quality and patient safety by:
(a) Collaborating with the Agency for Healthcare Research and Quality, the Centers for Medicare and Medicaid Ser-

vices, the Joint Commission, the National Committee for Quality Assurance, the National Quality Forum, and other data measurement, collection, cataloguing, and reporting agencies to evaluate changes in the performance of health professionals and the need for CPD in the improvement of patient care and safety; and

(b) Involving patients and consumers in CPD by using patient-reported measures and encouraging transparency to the public about performance of health care professionals.

DISSEMINATION OF CPD

In a comprehensive CPD system, proven techniques and methods would be identified and disseminated systematically to provide the greatest benefit for the investment. Mechanisms for spreading effective learning methods could take a number of forms. Descriptive reports detailing these methods could be distributed widely to CPD providers and health professionals interested in advancing training. Alternatively, effective CPD methods could be taught by qualified CPD providers to other providers. This would require a much more coordinated effort of training and evaluation than currently exists among CPD policy makers, planners, and evaluators, but such coordination would greatly facilitate the dissemination of CPD advances and eventually be of great benefit to patients and clinicians.

With a framework of CPD research and practice improvement, CPD providers will progressively increase their adherence to evidence-based CPD and surveillance data and contribute knowledge regarding CPD, improvement, and patient safety. An innovative e-health infrastructure can provide this opportunity through a variety of methods. For example, multimethod educational materials and electronic newsletters could support just-in-time learning; social networking environments such as Facebook and Twitter could promote tacit knowledge acquisition and co-creation of clinical knowledge, increasing opportunities to engage in electronic communities of practice. Simulations could also be used to train individuals and teams in disease management techniques. As technology advances, so, too, do the opportunities for e-learning.

ENHANCING THE PROFESSION OF CONTINUING
PROFESSIONAL DEVELOPMENT

In a better CPD system, schools, universities, and colleges would offer professional degrees or certificates with curricula designed to dramatically improve health professions education. Continuous learning—a much more dynamic approach to evidence development and application—would take full advantage of newer information technology to implement innovations. Programs and institutions dedicated to continuous learning and health care improvement would help the CPD system develop by providing a stable infrastructure and learning environment. Such institutions would house faculty expert in CPD. It is conceivable that many health professionals would want to learn in a specialized institution dedicated to developing comprehensive and integrated CPD programs, rather than collecting credits in a piecemeal and disjointed fashion. If these CPD programs were structured to provide premier educational opportunities, the professional drive to achieve excellence would likely also spur health professionals to enroll. Further, involvement in a community of professional learners and teachers to help individual practitioners advance would be a strong incentive for clinician enrollment, especially if the knowledge and skills they gained could be tied to improving the economics of their practice and improving the value of their care. As centers of CPD activity and scholarship, these institutions would be ideal vehicles to pilot-test and assess effective CPD curricula by providing reliable contexts for implementation and evaluation. Additionally, institutional structures for CPD could provide new levels of visibility and accountability for CPD and its resultant outcomes for learning, although health professionals would be responsible for their own learning and performance outcomes.

Current providers of CPD represent a resource for advancing CPD. CPD providers are skilled in needs assessment, instructional design, and program evaluation. Their roles as educators and mediators of health care quality improvement are critical but would be enhanced in a more effective CPD system, potentially leading to less variability, rational assessment standards for CPD pedagogy, and greater accountability. Ensuring that CPD providers receive access to quality data should improve the ability of assessment, education, and evaluative activities to influence the quality of care. Precision of research and evaluation also should improve with the development and availability of more valid and reliable outcome measures. CPD providers could also assume an important role in disseminating advances in CPD learning methods. Finally, like any group of professionals, CPD providers need to be held accountable to an ethical standard that best protects against conflicts of interest within the CPD system. These changes would bolster the value of providers, increase their motivation to improve instruction, and accelerate advances in CPD.

PUBLIC INVOLVEMENT AND ACCOUNTABILITY

Patients and consumers must be partners in a high-performing CPD system that promotes a culture of quality and patient safety. Transparency to the public and direct patient feedback and communication to health professionals foster a culture of accountability and purposeful learning. Patient input through patient-reported measures in research or by simply asking patients how quality of care could be improved are two ways to promote public involvement in CPD. Oversight systems should prioritize public accountability. Finally, efforts should be made to educate the public about CPD as the major mechanism for maintaining health professionals' competence. The health care system should adjust to shortcomings in the CPD system to assure the public of health professionals' competence.

CONCLUSIONS

Imagine a health care system with the ability to rapidly adapt to the needs of patients, health professionals, and institutions through a shared commitment to CPD and high quality patient care. Imagine a health care system in which everyone is a learner, supported on the arc of professional development with knowledge of tailored learning goals, the tools to meet and surpass those goals, and a community of other learners with whom to share the process. A comprehensive CPD system would transform this vision of professional learning into reality. To attain this goal, a new set of resources needs to be brought to bear, including a new scientific foundation for CPD, measures to assess the progress that CPD achieves, health information technology to spark faster transmission of data and facilitate learning activities, exchange of effective professional learning tools, interprofessional CPD programs, and a clear understanding among all stakeholders of the value proposition for CPD. Suffused throughout a better system must be a culture of public accountability, professionalism, and appreciation for the value of innovations in professional development, which will impel the system to better fulfill its aims. The recommended Continuing Professional Development

Institute (CPDI) is needed to drive these necessary improvements in CPD. Through guidance and coordination of efforts at these various levels, the CPDI can help the current system evolve into an improved system of effective continuing professional development to benefit practitioners, patients, and the public good.

REFERENCES

Cook, D. A., A. J. Levinson, S. Garside, D. M. Dupras, P. J. Erwin, and V. M. Montori. 2008. Internet-based learning in the health professions: A meta-analysis. *Journal of the American Medical Association* 300(10):1181-1196.

Davis, D., M. A. O'Brien, N. Freemantle, F. M. Wolf, P. Mazmanian, and A. Taylor-Vaisey. 1999. Impact of formal continuing medical education: Do conferences, workshops, rounds, and other traditional continuing education activities change physician behavior or health care outcomes? *Journal of the American Medical Association* 282(9):867-874.

Davis, D. A., P. E. Mazmanian, M. Fordis, R. Van Harrison, K. E. Thorpe, and L. Perrier. 2006. Accuracy of physician self-assessment compared with observed measures of competence: A systematic review. *Journal of the American Medical Association* 296(9):1094-1102.

Fordis, M., J. E. King, C. M. Ballantyne, P. H. Jones, K. H. Schneider, S. J. Spann, S. B. Greenberg, and A. J. Greisinger. 2005. Comparison of the instructional efficacy of Internet-based CME with live interactive CME workshops: A randomized controlled trial. *Journal of the American Medical Association* 294(9):1043-1051.

IOM (Institute of Medicine). 2003. *Health professions education: A bridge to quality.* Washington, DC: The National Academies Press.

Jackson, M. J., H. A. Gallis, S. C. Gilman, M. Grossman, G. B. Holzman, D. Marquis, and S. Trusky. 2007. The need for specialty curricula based on core competencies: A white paper of the Conjoint Committee on Continuing Medical Education. *Journal of Continuing Education in the Health Professions* 27(2):124-128.

Marinopoulos, S. S., T. Dorman, N. Ratanawongsa, L. M. Wilson, B. H. Ashar, J. L. Magaziner, R. G. Miller, P. A. Thomas, G. P. Prokopowicz, R. Qayyum, and E. B. Bass. 2007. *Effectiveness of continuing medical education.* Evidence report/technology assessment no. 149. Rockville, MD: Agency for Healthcare Research and Quality.

Miller, S. H., J. N. Thompson, P. E. Mazmanian, A. Aparicio, D. Davis, B. Spivey, and N. Kahn. 2008. Continuing medical education, professional development, and requirements for medical licensure: A white paper of the Conjoint Committee on Continuing Medical Education. *Journal of Continuing Education in the Health Professions* 28(2):95-98.

Moore, D. E., J. S. Green, and H. A. Gallis. 2009. Achieving desired results and improved outcomes: Integrating planning and assessment throughout learning activities. *Journal of Continuing Education in the Health Professions* 29(1):1-15.

Ratanawongsa, N., P. A. Thomas, S. S. Marinopoulos, T. Dorman, L. M. Wilson, B. H. Ashar, R. G. Miller, G. P. Prokopowicz, R. Qayyum, and E. B. Bass. 2008. The reported validity and reliability of methods for evaluating continuing medical education: A systematic review. *Academic Medicine* 83(3):274-283.

Reeves, S., M. Zwarenstein, J. Goldman, H. Barr, D. Freeth, M. Hammick, and I. Koppel. 2009. Interprofessional education: Effects on professional practice and health care outcomes. *Cochrane Database of Systematic Reviews* 23(1).

Spivey, B. E. 2005. Continuing medical education in the United States: Why it needs reform and how we propose to accomplish it. *Journal of Continuing Education in the Health Professions* 25(3):134-143.

6

Function and Structure of a Continuing Professional Development Institute

To achieve the goals of a new culture of continuing professional development (CPD), the recommended Continuing Professional Development Institute (CPDI) must be structured to advance continuing education (CE). Four areas in particular are fundamental to the scope of the recommended CPDI: advancing the science of CPD, data collection and dissemination, regulation, and financing. Furthermore, because one of the motivations for the CPDI is to promote collaboration across state and disciplinary lines, it should be guided by the principles of transparency (so that all stakeholders can participate and understand the results), independence (so that no organization dominates), use of best evidence (to convince diverse stakeholders of the CPDI's value), and analysis of the practitioner's experience as a professional development tool (to broaden the scope of CE). This chapter considers establishing the basic function and structure of the CPDI—and of the planning committee that will begin the process of consensus building and recommend the characteristics and operation of the CPDI in much greater detail than can be addressed in this report.

FUNCTION

Scientific Foundations of Continuing Professional Development

Congruent with the overall purpose of the CPDI, a research agenda should be developed that has collaboration and integration as its guiding principles, with the goal of enhancing knowledge of continuing professional development and ultimately improving patients' health outcomes. Research efforts should be developed through the collaboration of all individuals and organizations that conduct CPD, receive CPD, and benefit from CPD research, including the public. To support professional learning and development aimed at improving patient outcomes, research should inform practice, and practice should inform research by translating advances in medical knowledge and techniques into clinical practice much more quickly than now occurs.

CPD research should build knowledge about the theory of professional development, the methods used for CPD, and the measurements taken—all as related to the improvement of patient care quality, safety, and value. Other disciplines that are relevant and ought to be integrated into CPD research include adult education, organizational change, psychology, sociology, and systems engineering. These disciplines can shed light on behavior change in complex systems and help evaluate the impact of educational interventions on health outcomes.

Role of the CPDI in Research

The CPDI should develop the research agenda by establishing a comprehensive, collaborative research structure or center that coordinates CPD research and theory. It will also address its linkages to quality improvement, professional learning, and individual professional career advancement, system performance, and appropriate measurement. To hold the CPDI accountable for the development of a research agenda, the Secretary of the Department of Health and Human Services (the Secretary) should periodically monitor the CPDI's progress.

The CPDI is intended not to be a replacement for current research but to involve current researchers in creating a better system. Thus, the CPDI should serve a collaborating and convening function to foster a more comprehensive and integrated research structure. The focus on research that supports innovation, greater sources of funding, and improved patient care is incentive for researchers to participate in this effort. As part of a convening role, the CPDI would build consensus on research directions, set standards, and support the development and strengthening of research methods and the research workforce itself. Determining the success of these efforts will require developing measures and evaluation tool kits for research on knowledge, performance, outcomes, and gaps.

The CPDI should promote interdisciplinary and interprofessional research to integrate research being conducted in all health professions, other areas of health care (e.g., quality improvement, information technology, management and policy), and other relevant disciplines (e.g., adult learning, systems improvement). As noted in Chapter 5, other countries leading in CPD research could also be valuable collaborators. Best practices and theories may be gleaned from nonhealth-related industries, such as accounting, education, engineering, law, and transportation (see Appendix D).

Current funders of pertinent research will continue to solicit proposals and to award research grants; however, coordinating research areas with other organizations via the CPDI can enable funders to target their funds more effectively. Such collaboration could result in a CPDI that pioneers new, more effective forms of inquiry that would build on current methods. The CPDI should periodically identify gap areas, solicit proposals, and fund research to fill these gaps.

The National Quality Forum (NQF) is a model for a networking function that is similar to the objectives of the CPDI—i.e., providing an environment for researchers, professional societies, stakeholder organizations, and the government to learn from each other and exchange needs and desires to further the research agenda. Such a learning network would mirror the breadth of the CPDI and include the broad spectrum of researchers (from novice to expert), clinicians, and educators in all settings.

Science of CPD

The science of CPD must be considered along with research on CPD effectiveness. The science of CPD includes the theories and assumptions on which hypotheses and models of learning are developed. These theory-based frameworks are fundamental for formulating strong research questions. Inquiry into the science of CPD must include the science of measurement and the science of evaluation.

Both quantitative and qualitative methods can be applied to understanding the CPD continuum. For example, randomized controlled trials may not be appropriate for determining whether clinical guidelines change clinician behavior; instead this may require multimethod research approaches (Goering and Streiner, 1996; Morgan, 1998). The biological and social sciences should be used to foster the integration of different disciplines and professions. A multimethod approach has potential to strengthen the evidence for CPD.

Just as only appropriate methods should be used to study particular kinds of research questions, only appropriate educational methods should be used to understand and verify different needs and outcomes. An inventory of measurement instruments to evaluate the effectiveness and efficiency of CPD should be developed to support the broad application of validated measures.

> **Recommendation 4: The Continuing Professional Development Institute should lead efforts to improve the underlying scientific foundation of CPD to enhance the knowledge and performance of health professionals and patient outcomes by:**
> **(a) Integrating appropriate methods and findings from existing research in a variety of disciplines and professions,**
> **(b) Generating research directions that advance understanding and application of new CPD solutions to problems associated with patient and population health status,**
> **(c) Transform new knowledge pertinent to CPD into tools and methods for increasing the success of efforts to improve patient health, and**
> **(d) Promoting the development of an inventory of measurement instruments that can be used to evaluate the effectiveness and efficiency of CPD.**

Data Collection and Dissemination

As the underpinnings of research, data are the basis for informed decision making. Accurate and reliable data often require measurement validation and audit. Current continuing education efforts typically suffer from a lack of high quality data on which to base decisions and do not adequately couple theory and measurement. The result has been that decisions about continuing education and professional development are not always based on evidence. More importantly, no coordinated effort exists to systematically collect these data, yielding concentrated areas of research that are not necessarily connected to one another.

To advance CPD research and support evidence-based decision making, the CPDI should ensure that data are collected, analyzed, and publicly reported to allow for the evaluation of CPD methods and providers. These data ought to also clarify and build knowledge about linkages between CPD, better patient care, and better performance of health care systems. Specifically, data should help determine what effectively influences the health professional's capacity to meet the goals described by the Institute of Medicine (IOM) to deliver safe, effective, patient-centered, timely, efficient, and equitable health care services (IOM, 2001). Collection of such data will require a significant investment of time and resources but is fundamental to creating an effective CPD system. Data should facilitate the alignment of good learning and good health care and should identify the skills required to meet educational needs and choose the appropriate tools to teach and assess the required skills.

At the systems level, it will be critical to collect and evaluate data on the cost of CPD and its financing to better understand the value and create a business case for specific CPD activities. These analyses are essential for making decisions about how CPD resources should be invested. Collection of more robust and comprehensive data on CPD would provide a strong evidence-base on which to build through aggregation at the individual professional level, organizational level, and systems level.

The CPDI's role as a central convener would entail endorsing educational measures, determining the data to be collected and reported, identifying the manner in which they are reported, and creating a coordinated network to develop a robust data system that advances current efforts and best practices. These roles can be fulfilled only if the CPDI works with interdisciplinary researchers and health professionals, while serving as a central resource. Researchers in the service and academic communities should continue to develop and store data but, when appropriate, should offer to share data when requested by the CPDI (see Box 6-1).

The approaches used by the quality improvement field provide a good analogy for how to collect and disseminate data. Organizations such as the Agency for Healthcare Research and Quality, the Centers for Medicare and Medicaid Services, The Joint Commission, the National Committee for Quality Assurance, and the National Quality Forum, among others, have distinct roles in data measurement, collection, and reporting. Partnership between CPD organizations and organizations whose purpose is to improve quality and patient safety would provide benefits beyond applying lessons learned. The relationship between continuing professional development and quality improvement suggests that the communities would have overlapping needs for performance measurement standards, data collection and reporting, and ways of gathering and offering feed-

---

BOX 6-1
Trusted Agent Model:
Compiling Evidence to Support CPD

Large amounts of data exist on all physicians, but they are stored in different data repositories. Records of attendance and performance in medical school, residency, board examinations, board certification status, licensing, attendance at continuing medical education activities, and case logs and portfolios of clinical and educational experiences are housed separately. The application process for state licensure is tedious and time consuming—requiring months to verify each primary source—and is repeated each time a physician seeks to be credentialed or licensed, adding substantial burden and expense for the physician and for the state board and/or hospital.

The Trusted Agent Model was developed by the National Board of Medical Examiners (NBME) Center for Innovation. It is an example of a data-sharing infrastructure that compiles evidence of a physician's credentials and learning. Data are compiled from several sources (trusted agents) and, after use, can be destroyed without affecting the original data sources. The Trusted Agent Model was tested in a joint demonstration project of 2,810 applicants conducted by the NBME and the Federation of State Medical Boards in Kentucky, New Hampshire, and Ohio, requiring agreement with the regulatory bodies and permission by applicants to release the data. Instead of months, physician credentials were verified in *8 seconds*.

The Trusted Agent concept has yet to be tested as an interactive professional development tool; however, when coupled with learning portfolios, it could enable documentation of learning from diverse sources for any desired use, including public transparency. Conceivably, the CPDI could deploy the Trusted Agent Model or similar concepts across health professions to foster ongoing professional development, document clinical and learning experiences, identify interprofessional learning experiences and team development, and provide the public with data about the types of patients a health professional team sees and its clinical and educational outcomes. Reduction in the burden and costs associated with documenting health professional credentials could be substantial.

---

back on health care professionals' performance. The Office of the National Coordinator for Health Information Technology should be leveraged as a partner toward collection of such data and can help develop standardized learning portfolios as a tool for collecting common data on professionals across the country.

Recommendation 5: The Continuing Professional Development Institute should enhance the collection of data to enable evaluation and assessment of CPD at the individual, team,

organizational, system, and national levels. Efforts should include:

(a) Relating quality improvement data to CPD, and
(b) Collaborating with the Office of the National Coordinator for Health Information Technology in developing national standardized learning portfolios to enhance the understanding of the linkages between educational interventions, skill acquisition, and improvement of patient care.

Regulation

The recommendation to create the CPDI is motivated in part by a significant need to improve the licensure, certification, and credentialing of health professionals by the various health professions, and to improve the process of accreditation of continuing education providers. The institute should focus first on improving accreditation. Accreditation discerns and publicly recognizes that a CPD provider meets minimum standards of quality. As discussed in Chapter 3, the committee is not proposing that responsibility be given to different accreditors but that accreditation systems be modified to address the entire continuum of CPD and to focus more on discerning, recognizing, and improving professionals' competence and performance. Such a system would allow health professionals to better understand how to improve their practices. Innovation toward these ends requires cooperation from current accreditors to drive change in the accreditation system toward learner-driven CPD.

In most cases, the accreditation and certification processes have been the responsibility of the professions themselves. For the majority of health professions, certification is administered at the national level. Accreditation of CE programs occurs at both the national and the state levels, largely under the direction of professional societies. Accreditation offers a particularly interesting model, where national accreditation bodies can sometimes set standards and accredit the state societies, which in turn sanction local CE providers. The dual system of national and state accreditation should be consolidated to the extent possible. Accreditors tend to accredit providers of educational programs rather than the programs themselves, distancing the accreditors from the improvement of patient care. Today, it is possible to accredit tools, such as individual learning portfolios, which are much more tightly linked to the health professional's practice.

Professional societies that function as regulators (e.g., American Medical Association, American Dental Association, National Council for Therapeutic Recreation Certification, the National League of

Nursing) ordinarily maintain knowledge and expertise sufficient to conduct various monitoring tasks, but it is outside their scope to conduct rigorous research for improvement or to explain causal relationships of accreditation, credit, certification, licensure, continuing education, and improved quality of care. There is a need for coordination and collaboration among regulators and researchers, both within the same profession and among professions, to explore and test the relationships of regulation to more effective continuing education and health care. Cross-disciplinary regulatory mechanisms will become increasingly important with a greater focus by the system on interprofessional education. The committee concludes that the CPDI should work with current regulatory bodies to develop regulatory policies and establish national standards for all health professions. The CPDI should, in effect, develop standards for and accredit the accrediting bodies.

Soon after the CPDI is established, it should establish a collaborative process for gathering perspectives from all appropriate stakeholders through public hearings and other methods of due process to set national, interprofessional standards for accreditation. In the longer term, a process will be needed to evaluate and update the standards and continually monitor the accreditors. The role of the CPDI should periodically be reassessed to determine whether there is a proper balance between government regulation and professional self-regulation.

> **Recommendation 6: The Continuing Professional Development Institute should work with stakeholders to develop national standards for regulation of CPD. The CPDI should set standards for regulatory bodies across the health professions for licensure, certification, credentialing, and accreditation.**

Improved CPD Financing

The CPDI should have as a major responsibility identifying and acquiring more stable sources of financing to fund a broad-based, comprehensive CPD system. The issues of bias and conflicts of interest arise when discussing who should fund CPD activities and research (Steinbrook, 2005, 2008). The committee believes that all CPD funding should align with the committee's defined purposes for CPD—improved quality of care and patient safety. All funders whose primary goal is not improved quality of care and patient safety should be restricted from providing either financial or in-kind support to CPD, although it is understood that not all commercial funding is conflicted and that there may be many other conflicted sources that do not involve commercial sources.

To help the CPDI more rapidly incorporate this into its accreditation standards, the planning committee will need to develop guiding principles to address conflicts of interest. These principles should build on the guidelines already developed on conflict of interest, some of which have been set forth by organizations and partnerships such as the Accreditation Council for Continuing Medical Education (ACCME) and the Pharmaceutical Research and Manufacturers Association (PhRMA), and should build on the work of an IOM report on conflict of interest (ACCME, 2006; IOM, 2009; PhRMA, 2008). These will make a good starting point for the CPDI to establish standardized guidelines on conflicted sources of funding for CPD at the national level for all professions. The planning committee may determine that investments from conflicted sources may still be used if directed in specific ways (e.g., pooling money, with the CPDI or some other neutral body having discretion over how it is spent).

Implementation of the proposed restrictions on conflicted funding could mean that the sources of a sizable amount of current funds may no longer be able to invest in the CPDI and improved CPD system. In the absence of evidence, there is very likely enough money in the current system to support a better one, given the proposed changes in the scope of CPD programs and the opportunities to reduce the waste and inefficiencies documented in Chapter 3.

Recommendation 7: The Continuing Professional Development Institute should analyze the sources and adequacy of funding for CPD, develop a sustainable business model free from conflicts of interest, and promote the use of CPD to improve quality and patient safety.

STRUCTURE OF A CONTINUING PROFESSIONAL DEVELOPMENT INSTITUTE

The following section outlines the structure this IOM committee has envisioned for the Continuing Professional Development Institute (see Figure 6-1).

The Planning Committee

As recommended in Chapter 4, a planning committee should be commissioned with the specific tasks of outlining the CPDI's

124

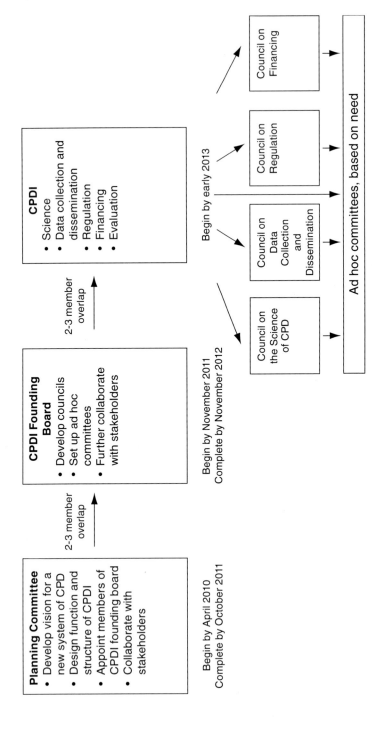

Planning Committee
- Develop vision for a new system of CPD
- Design function and structure of CPDI
- Appoint members of CPDI founding board
- Collaborate with stakeholders

Begin by April 2010
Complete by October 2011

2-3 member overlap

CPDI Founding Board
- Develop councils
- Set up ad hoc committees
- Further collaborate with stakeholders

Begin by November 2011
Complete by November 2012

2-3 member overlap

CPDI
- Science
- Data collection and dissemination
- Regulation
- Financing
- Evaluation

Council on the Science of CPD

Council on Data Collection and Dissemination

Council on Regulation

Council on Financing

Begin by early 2013

Ad hoc committees, based on need

FIGURE 6-1 Suggested process for the development of a CPDI.

scope of work, developing the CPDI's governance model, identifying sources of financial stability for the CPDI, and identifying and managing relationships with new and current stakeholders. This IOM committee believes that the planning committee ought to operate under four principles:

- The planning committee should be held accountable by the public and the Secretary;
- The planning committee should be competency-based, flexible, and nimble;
- The planning committee should broadly communicate with, and gather input from, the rest of the field (e.g., health professions, accreditors, CPD providers, licensing bodies), but only planning committee members should receive voting rights; and
- The planning committee should use consensus building, not parliamentary procedure, to manage its operations.

In designing the CPDI as a public-private partnership, the planning committee should also not be solely public or solely private. The quality of professionals' performance, which is the focus of CPD, is currently largely the responsibility of the professions and the state agencies that provide licensure, so that embedding the planning committee in a federal agency would not be appropriate. However, no professional organization or group of organizations has the ability or authority currently to develop the collaborative and integrative efforts the committee believes necessary for CPD. Thus, the planning committee should be funded by contracts and grants from the government and private foundations to enable funding for staff and travel.

Membership

The two main options for the composition of the planning committee are a representational structure and a competency-based structure. Appendix B lists the categories of health care practitioner and technical occupations as identified by the Bureau of Labor Statistics (U.S. Bureau of Labor Statistics, 2008). Professions requiring baccalaureate or higher degrees should be recognized as stakeholders of the CPDI. Although representation from each profession or each category of professions would be ideal in terms of hearing from all perspectives, requiring different representation from all or a large majority of the 54 professions listed in Table B-1 would result in a planning committee that is too large to function; 13 to 15 members is a more effective size. Additionally, those who conduct research, those who sponsor CPD activities, and those who benefit from CPD are also stakeholders whose perspectives need to be considered. The planning committee should also have the ability to adapt to emerging realities without undue influence of some members or other stakeholders. The committee therefore concludes that a representational structure would not best serve the goals of the planning committee, and its members should instead be chosen on the basis of competency.

Competencies that the committee believes are important to include on the planning committee are listed in Box 6-2. Members may be knowledgeable in more than one of the identified areas; each area should be represented more than once, if possible. Given the planning committee's significant role in shaping the future of CPD and building relationships with stakeholders, it is important for all planning committee members to be thought leaders in their respective fields, have experience in leading change and improvement, and have some level of experience in interprofessional learning. Planning committee membership should at a minimum include practicing professionals and individuals with expertise in government and CPD research. The need to be mindful of historically underrepresented groups also applies to the planning committee membership. The planning committee chair should be an executive manager with a record of success in setting and implementing visions and building consensus. All members, including the chair, should be appointed by the Secretary of the Department of Health and Human Services, in consultation with other federal departments.

Procedures

The planning committee should operate on the principle of *intelligent* consensus building. Operations should therefore not be driven by parliamentary procedure, where the views of individuals often serve the purpose of bias and separation.

The planning committee must foster relationships with other stakeholders. Operating under the principles of transparency, the planning committee should hold public hearings to gather a more diverse set of opinions in its decision-making processes. However, only planning committee members would vote.

A report should be delivered to the Secretary detailing the outcomes of its deliberations.

BOX 6-2
Competencies for Planning Committee Membership

A competency-based committee formed to plan the CPDI should consist of members who (1) are considered thought leaders in their respective fields, (2) have experience in leading change and improvement, and (3) have experience in interprofessional learning. At a minimum, membership should include practicing health professionals and individuals with expertise in government and CPD research. Competencies that ought to be represented on the planning committee are listed alphabetically below.

- Accreditation, certification, and licensing
- Adult learning and clinical education, including design and evaluation of CPD methods
- Care coordination and team training
- Economics
- Ethics and conflicts of interest
- Health care reform
- International perspective
- Measurement
- Microsystem and macrosystem experiences
- Payer, not from a federal perspective
- Quality improvement, focusing on the science and techniques of improvement
- State perspective with an understanding of the state governments' roles in licensure

---

Continuing Professional Development Institute

The IOM committee based its ideas for the CPDI on the notion that the CPDI's vision statement should be "supporting competent clinicians for quality patient care." To fulfill this vision, the mission of the CPDI should be to coordinate and integrate efforts of all stakeholders to enhance professional development for the purpose of improving health care quality and patient safety. Upon its development, the CPDI founding board should adopt its own vision statement, while keeping in mind the original intents.

Board

The board of directors is the key body that approves the mission, vision, and goals of an organization. The CPDI board should view its role as laying the foundation for a culture of learning to achieve high quality, safe health care. Like the planning committee and for the same reasons, it should be competency-based, with competencies similar to those of the planning committee; however, the planning committee should make the final determination of the exact competencies required. It may wish to consider including a member of the public. Membership size and structure of the founding board should also be determined by the planning committee. To facilitate the transition from planning committee to CPDI, some members of the planning committee should serve on the founding board (see Figure 5-1). Upon development of a more permanent structure, board members should rotate in an overlapping manner.

Operating Structure

With such a broad mission of coordinating and integrating the CPD efforts of all stakeholders, many organizations and categories of individuals should be included in the operations of the CPDI. A limitation to a competency-based board is that more stakeholders exist than can reasonably sit on a board. Therefore, a structure that adopts the use of standing councils and analogous methods, such as ad hoc committees, seems necessary to incorporate the perspectives of a broad group of stakeholders. The rest of this report is written with the expectation that standing councils will be created for each of the CPDI's four major responsibilities: science of CPD, data collection and dissemination, regulation, and financing (see Figure 6-1). Councils are envisioned to be relatively small in size, with the board determining council membership. The primary purpose of the councils would be to provide transparency through fair and equitable processes and advise the board on complex issues. The secondary purpose would be to gather stakeholder groups with specific expertise so that the board's decisions will be based on a broader perspective. The appropriate topics for councils will likely change as the CPD system develops, so the board will need to periodically reevaluate what councils should exist. Ad hoc committees, on the other hand, would be convened to gather public opinion on a specific identified need and would disband after completing its work. For example, a problem-focused committee might be established to advise on how to operationalize team-based learning.

The founding board should consider including a broad set of voices on the councils and ad hoc committees. The voices of patients are critical and should not be excluded. Additionally, the breadth of stakeholders should also incorporate the quality improvement community. Together, councils and ad hoc committees would provide a process for the voices of those not on the board to be heard, for issues to be debated, and for facilitation of decision making. Other avenues for stakeholder input should continuously be considered and developed, as deemed necessary by the board. Like the CPDI in general, these councils and ad hoc committees should work toward the goal of improving quality and patient safety.

Public-Private Partnership

The CPDI is envisioned to be an independent body with membership and financing from both the public and the private sectors. This structure allows for the planning committee to operate without undue influences from individual stakeholders, including federal and state governments, professional organizations, and industry alike.

Currently, no organization within continuing education or CPD in the United States has the ability or authority to bring together all stakeholders. The federal government, through the Secretary of Health and Human Services, is in the best position to provide initial oversight and serve as the locus for coordination toward development of the CPDI. After formation of the CPDI, the Secretary or any other federal department such as the Department of Education would not have any specific formal role, unless one is identified and recommended by the planning committee. Oversight and coordination should eventually be transferred back to the professions when it becomes clear that the government no longer needs to serve in a leadership and coordinating role, as determined by the CPDI board.

As with the planning committee, the CPDI should be sponsored by and receive funding from both government and private foundations. Establishment and maintenance of learning portfolios offers a source of service revenue to support the institute's work over the long term. Organizational membership fees should be discouraged because board and council members would then be less independent. Determination of the size of the CPDI's budget depends on its exact functions and breadth, so it will be the planning committee's job to estimate and project a budget for the CPDI once it has determined the details of those elements. The planning committee should provide guidance for long-term funding for the CPDI and for ensuring that the acceptance of funds from conflicted sources does not bias the work of the CPDI.

Proposed Activities

Communications and dissemination of achievements are necessary components for the growth of the CPDI and acceptance of
its role by all stakeholders. Lessons learned, decisions made, and
research findings must be shared widely. The CPDI would need
adequate latitude from not only its board but also its stakeholders
to constantly adapt, allowing it to function as a learning system.
Without broad communication, the goals of collaboration and integration cannot be met. A strong communications and dissemination
plan should therefore be a core function of the CPDI. For example,
the research arm of the CPDI could develop and widely distribute a
periodic (e.g., quarterly) consensus document about the state of the
art of CPD in relation to specific research areas.

Evaluation is also a fundamental component of an institute.
Measures of success should be developed by the planning committee to monitor the CPDI's activities and progress. Feedback on the
CPDI's activities is critical to continuously improving professional
development with the aim of better health outcomes.

REFERENCES

ACCME (Accreditation Council for Continuing Medical Education). 2006. *ACCME
  essential areas and their elements: Updated decision-making criteria relevant to the essential areas and elements.* Chicago, IL: ACCME.
Goering, P. N., and D. L. Streiner. 1996. Reconcilable differences: The marriage of
  qualitative and quantitative methods. *Canadian Journal of Psychiatry* 41(8):491-
  497.
IOM (Institute of Medicine). 2001. *Crossing the quality chasm: A new health system for
  the 21st century.* Washington, DC: National Academy Press.
———. 2009. *Conflict of interest in medical research, education, and practice.* Washington,
  DC: The National Academies Press.
Morgan, D. L. 1998. Practical strategies for combining qualitative and quantitative
  methods: Applications to health research. *Qualitative Health Research* 8(3):362-
  376.
PhRMA (Pharmaceutical Research and Manufacturers of America). 2008. *Code on
  interactions with healthcare professionals.* Washington, DC: PhRMA.
Steinbrook, R. 2005. Commercial support and continuing medical education. *New
  England Journal of Medicine* 352(6):534-535.
———. 2008. Financial support of continuing medical education. *Journal of the American Medical Association* 299(9):1060-1062.
U.S. Bureau of Labor Statistics. 2008. *Occupational outlook handbook, 2008-09 edition.*
  Washington, DC: U.S. Bureau of Labor Statistics.

7

Implementation, Research, and Evaluation

This chapter provides some guidance on implementation of the Continuing Professional Development Institute (CPDI), suggests a framework for research on continuing professional development (CPD), and offers ways to assess the CPDI.

IMPLEMENTATION

Creating a New Culture

The first step toward establishing the CPDI will be to begin the development of an environment and infrastructure that support life-long learning and interprofessional education. Buy-in and general agreement will be needed from stakeholders at all levels to change their own cultures and to alter current continuing education (CE) practices.

Pivotal to such a major culture change is the critical role of leadership in communicating a compelling vision, aligning incentives and accountabilities, and establishing a collaborative and engaged management team to create the infrastructure necessary to improve and support the evolution of the CPDI. Management must also be attentive to its own development and preparation to success-fully lead the cultural change. For example, within hospitals and academic health centers, learning could be fostered through the appointment of a chief learning officer who would design and oversee a system of interprofessional, team-based learning that focuses on the delivery of evidence-based health care. Health professionals themselves, as well as teachers of CPD and other stakeholders, will need to reorient their ideas of the necessity and purpose for CPD activities and the roles they will have to play as continuous learners in order to consistently deliver the best possible care.

Concentrated efforts to begin this movement are needed to prevent further delays in improving health care quality and safety. To this end, the planning committee should cultivate relationships with relevant stakeholders, who in turn need to consider how they can best support the continuous development of the health care workforce. The scope of relevant stakeholders is broader than those directly involved in the learning of the U.S. health professions workforce. The United States can learn from the positive and negative experiences of other countries (e.g., Canada, European Union, United Kingdom) that have systems and structures in place to direct professional development, thus shortening the lead time needed to implement a U.S. CPD system (see Appendix C). International cooperation is a source of mutual learning, and initially the CPDI would likely learn from the best practices of other countries. Once a comprehensive CPD system is in place in the United States, the CPDI would be able to be an active member of the global CPD community by sharing its lessons learned.

Best practices could also be learned from and shared with other industries, such as engineering and teaching, which also require continuing education to assure the public of professionals' competence (see Appendix D). While the content must reflect the needs of the different industries, strategies for encouraging behavior change and learning are applicable across industries. The CPDI could benefit itself and others by being an active part of a continued learning community that spans all industries for which continued learning and development are critical.

Development of the CPDI is an important step toward ensuring health professionals' capacity to provide high quality care, but it is only one part of improving the quality and safety of the larger health care system. A strong connection needs to be created between CPD for clinicians and quality improvement at the micro-, meso-, and macrosystem levels. The microsystem refers to the front line of care, the network of interdependent people, information, and technology working together to accomplish a specific aim (e.g., ambulatory pediatric clinic, labor and delivery room, inpatient unit). The mesosystem creates the environment for transformation and includes the resources, strategies, and measures to guide and track change. Mesosystems enable interdependent functioning of multiple microsystems and confront impediments to good patient care—for example, from poor information systems or from relationships that do not recognize true interdependence. The macrosystem sets a vision and goals to guide the micro- and mesosystems by providing an enabling context and leadership for change. Professional development strategies and alignment of incentives are fostered at the macrosystem level. They are a natural point of accountability for the care outcomes of a community (Nelson et al., 2007).

Interprofessional, Team-Based Care

A concept underlying the CPDI is that by bringing together diverse participants, it will support and advance the team-based nature of health care. Health care often requires coordination among multiple practitioners, both intraprofessionally and interprofessionally. Today, care is often not practiced in teams, not because teams are not useful or effective, but because people are not trained in such a fashion. As the health professions are increasingly recognized as interdependent, a new team-based culture will emerge. The professional environment will also change as patients become more active partners in their health care. To embody the principles of effective interprofessional education, the CPDI will need to pursue four goals:

1. Articulate a coherent rationale for implementing interprofessional continuing education,
2. Promote collaboration to achieve patient-centered aims,
3. Reconcile competing objectives between the professions in a way that is accepted by all of them, while reinforcing collaborative competence, and
4. Support the development of methods to recognize interprofessional activities in the credentialing of individual professions.

A number of interprofessional experiments in CPD have been developed, resulting in pockets of interprofessional programs. It is important that these experiences could be supported, built on, and expanded in clinical practices in settings such as integrated health care systems and academic health centers. Academic health centers would be particularly interesting, given their important roles in undergraduate and graduate education. Applying these principles to CPD will promote a unified educational framework, align communication, and share advances across all health professions.

>   **Recommendation 8: The Continuing Professional Development Institute should identify, recognize, and foster models of CPD that build knowledge about interprofessional team learning and collaboration.**

Regulation

The standing Council on Regulation ought to consider how it would best align the various regulatory processes with a broader view of CPD. Several regulatory bodies have announced nascent efforts to streamline some of their processes (ACCME, 2009); historically, similar initiatives have been neither frequent nor interprofessional. Interprofessional cooperation to enhance regulatory processes should be encouraged to the greatest extent possible to support development of comprehensive, team-based care. By encouraging and facilitating action by various regulatory bodies across states and professions to ensure the competence of all practitioners, the CPDI can promote the consistency and alignment of regulations. Policies to align regulatory efforts should be developed based on evidence, allowing for minimum standards to be set in areas such as the methods and amount of CPD necessary for optimal learning.

Processes to improve the coherence of regulations will need to take all stakeholders' perspectives into account. One promising approach, for example, is the development of model laws in state-based licensing. The process used by the National Association of Insurance Commissioners to develop model laws could be adapted to promote regulatory improvements at the level of individual states.

Disruptive innovations may be necessary to introduce positive change to the regulatory system. For example, in certification, the Council on Regulation could consider mandatory maintenance of certification programs for all health professions. A program of this nature could also be coupled with mandatory maintenance of licensure programs. These programs could help certification and licensure processes enhance practice performance and become better resources for the public. Maintenance of certification has become mandatory for physician specialties to ensure minimum levels of skill maintenance and competence (ABMS, 2009). This concept has not yet been adopted by all professions that grant certification. However, if minimum standards were applied across the health professions (given that different professions require different amounts of learning), the public could be ensured that all practitioners, despite their profession or specialty, have the ability to perform competently and to improve the safety and quality of health care. Similarly, the Federation of State Medical Boards has recently developed some guidance on maintenance of licensure programs to support physician commitment to lifelong learning (FSMB, 2008); these programs have yet to be implemented.

To catalyze a movement toward improved learning, the Council on Regulation will need to support disruptive innovations and might consider working with licensing bodies to depart from the traditional credit-based system to a more performance-based system. A credit-based system may fuel health professionals' indifference toward CPD by allowing a range of activities to count for continuing education that are not related to the maintenance or advancement of competence. A performance-based system, although harder to administer, would do just the opposite by ensuring that all health professionals maintain minimum levels of competence in their specialty areas. Such a system could provide leverage for the CPDI and licensing and certification bodies, anchoring CPD efforts in performance improvement.

Financing

The first challenge for the Council on Financing will be to stimulate the adoption of conflict-of-interest guidelines for all health professions to prohibit conflicted sources from funding CPD activities and CPD research. While many organizations at all levels of CPD have developed such guidance, no single industrywide standard exists for CPD. Although conflicted sources of funding more intensely permeate some professions than others, a single set of guidelines across the health professions would help protect the integrity of a CPD system. Additionally, the council will need to consider development of processes that would require CPD funders to declare their conflicts of interest to the institute.

Conflicted sources of funding can be reduced or eliminated only if there is a parallel effort to identify nonconflicted sources of funding for CPD and CPD research. This effort will need to involve a broad group of stakeholders and a reconsideration of how CPD is funded and the roles of employers and government in directly supporting CPD. By strengthening the link between professional development and patient outcomes, collaboration with groups such as the quality improvement community may lead to investments in

CPD that meet conflict of interest guidelines. A reconstitution of the mix of CPD funders or, at a minimum, diversification of funders that limits the financing from any one source may be necessary. For example, in the absence of conflicted sources of funding, academic health centers and health care organizations may provide greater levels of financial support, along with individual practitioners themselves, as discussed in Chapter 3. All models should be considered and assessed for the ability to strengthen CPD financing.

As discussed in Chapter 6, a small number of research gaps might be identified for funding from the CPDI. A central pool of money could be created to distribute funds to support this research and other activities deemed necessary by the CPDI that would otherwise not be funded. For example, one likely area for research is in analyzing data to determine the value proposition for CPD, and cost-benefit analyses should be performed. These calculations might not be of interest to professional societies, which would be more likely to sponsor research on particular CPD activities and learning methods. In the absence of an appropriate funder, the use of central funds could allow important research to move forward. The mechanisms and guidelines for creating such a system need to be considered by the planning committee and, in the beginning stages of the CPDI, the Council on Financing.

Another aspect of improving financing for CPD is the creation of incentives for CPD stakeholders to do the right thing. Both monetary and nonmonetary incentives could be designed to achieve the vision of a better CPD system. Nonmonetary incentives might include professional recognition and career advancement in the workplace.

RESEARCH

As discussed in Chapters 5 and 6, research is a core function of the CPDI and must be strengthened if truly effective advancements are to take place in CPD to discover what works where and to what degree. Research needs to be practical and to be based on practice needs. Coordination and communication systems should be facilitated by the Council on the Science of CPD. Because research relies on data, the council should be supported by the Council on Data Collection and Dissemination. The two councils should work together to advance research and the state of CPD.

Setting Priorities

In an inclusive, deliberative process, the CPDI should set national priorities on which research areas and topics should be funded. Doing so will require identification of criteria. The committee considered criteria used by other organizations to set priorities (see Table 7-1), including the Agency for Healthcare Research and

TABLE 7-1 Criteria Adopted by Select Organizations

Criteria	AHRQ	EPOC	HRSA	NPP	CPDI
Urgency of the problem	✓	✓			✓
Gaps in current knowledge		✓			✓
Opportunity to improve practice[a]	✓	✓			✓
Innovation in methods					✓
Ability to advance the science of CPD					✓
Appropriateness (priority population or condition)	✓				
Desirability of new research documentation	✓	✓			
Feasibility	✓				
Improve health outcomes[a]	✓		✓		
Improve delivery of effective health care services, quality of care provided		✓	✓		
Improve access to health care services			✓		
Eliminate harm, improve patient safety				✓	
Eradicate or eliminate disparities	✓		✓	✓	
Reduce disease burden				✓	
Remove waste				✓	

NOTE: The difference between CPDI criteria and those of other groups largely stems from the difference in each organization's purpose.

[a] AHRQ combines these criteria into one criterion, "potential value," that also includes the potential for significantly impacting health and reducing unnecessary burden (cost) on those with health care problems.

Quality (AHRQ), the Effective Practice and Organisation of Care (EPOC) Review Group, the Health Resources and Services Administration (HRSA), and the National Priorities Partnership (NPP).

Although AHRQ has no specific agencywide means of setting priorities, the AHRQ Effective Health Care Program aims to improve the quality, effectiveness, and efficiency of the health care delivery system by using systematic reviews when comparing the effectiveness and harms of different health care interventions (Slutsky et al., 2008). The program uses the following criteria: reviews must be relevant and timely, be objective and scientifically rigorous, be transparent and involve public participation, and set a priority list for topics to review, including conditions such as cancer, cardiovascular disease, and obesity (Slutsky et al., 2008; Whitlock et al., 2009).

EPOC is part of the Cochrane Collaboration[1] and specifically develops systematic reviews of interventions aiming to improve professional practice and the delivery of health care services, through continuing education, quality assurance, financial, organizational, and regulatory interventions. Much like AHRQ, EPOC as a whole does not have a specific set of priorities outlined at present; however, this is a future goal.[2] Its Norwegian satellite, however, does have specific criteria to use when setting priorities for its systematic reviews. It focuses specifically on interventions that are relevant to low- and middle-income countries; if the topic is of importance to a low- or middle-income country, a Cochrane-conducted systematic review could help to inform appropriate decisions about how to address this problem. Also, if a review has already been conducted on the specific topic, there has to be good reason to update or conduct a new review (EPOC, 2009).

HRSA aims to improve "access to health care services for people who are uninsured, isolated, or medically vulnerable," through activities such as providing health care services to vulnerable populations, training health professionals, and improving systems of care in rural parts of the United States (HRSA, 2009). HRSA's priorities seek to provide those who are uninsured, those who are under-

---

[1] "The Cochrane Collaboration is an international not-for-profit and independent organization, dedicated to making up-to-date, accurate information about the effects of health care readily available worldwide. It produces and disseminates systematic reviews of health care interventions and promotes the search for evidence in the form of clinical trials and other studies of interventions"; see http://www.cochrane.org/docs/descrip.htm.

[2] Personal communication with A. Mayhew, EPOC Managing Editor, April 23, 2009.

served, and those with special needs with access to health care services they otherwise would be unable to use (HRSA, 2005).

The NPP, convened by the National Quality Forum, is a collaborative effort of major national health care organizations that collectively influence every part of the health care system—both the private and the public sectors—including consumers, purchasers, quality alliances, health professionals and providers, insurers, government, accreditation and certification programs, and others (NPP, 2008). When setting its initial six priorities—patient and family engagement, population health, safety, care coordination, palliative and end-of-life care, and overuse—the NPP focused on high-leverage areas that would have the most immediate impact on reaching the goals of eliminating harm, eradicating health care disparities, reducing disease burden, and removing waste from the health care system. The NPP believes that such cross-cutting areas provide the greatest potential to substantially improve health and health care and to fundamentally change the U.S. health care delivery system.

Recognizing that these organizations developed criteria for specific purposes that are not identical to those of CPD research, the committee suggests the following five criteria as a basis for prioritizing CPD research: urgency of the problem, gaps in current knowledge, opportunity to improve practice, innovation in methods, and ability to advance the science of CPD. The criteria are all of equal importance.

- *Urgency of the problem.* The urgency of the problem being researched can be assessed at the individual, public, and population health levels, using various measures. At the individual level, measures may include severity of conditions, disease burden, and quality of life as a result of a given condition. At the public and population health levels, measures such as prevalence and cost could be used.
- *Gaps in current knowledge.* Research topics should also be prioritized according to whether they address gaps in current knowledge. Gaps should be identified by the CPDI in the areas of structure, process, and outcomes. Outcomes can be considered at the level of patients, practitioners, systems, and society. At the CPD provider level, gaps in knowledge occur in understanding the effectiveness and comparative effectiveness of various delivery methods (e.g., lectures, journals) as well as of CPD content (e.g., behavior change, performance improvement). Improvement in the state of CPD science requires continuous reassessment of research gaps.

- *Opportunity to improve practice.* A greater understanding is needed to bridge the gap between research and practice. Research should therefore be given higher priority if it is deemed to have the ability to improve the practical knowledge, skills, and attitudes of clinicians.
- *Innovation in methods.* Innovation is critical to making systems changes. With respect to CPD, researchers should be encouraged and rewarded for developing innovations in delivery methods and research methods. Research projects that provide new approaches and perspectives will be important in advancing CPD.
- *Ability to advance the science of CPD.* Research is needed to advance the science of CPD. The science of CPD includes the methods of studying CPD and its underlying theories and hypotheses.

The Council on the Science of CPD should consider the criteria described above when determining research areas and priorities. A coordinated research agenda could reduce unnecessary duplication of research with other programs, link with other fields in health care to broaden the research base, and provide more evidence on the availability of effective methods and best practices.

The planning committee should define a process for setting a research agenda, and an early task for the Council on the Science of CPD is to refine and implement that process. To determine who might set priorities, three nonexclusive options were considered: a broad set of professional groups and other stakeholders, a group similar to EPOC that would specifically focus on CPD, or the CPDI based on advice from the standing council. Since the purpose of a coordinated research agenda is to foster collaboration and integration, learners, experts, and facilitators should all be involved in agenda setting. Central planning is needed to develop a comprehensive research agenda and to reduce bias. For example, a research group similar to EPOC could be developed as a first step to produce systematic reviews examining topics related to CPD. Second, priorities could be set by researchers across professions. Finally, the committee considered the potential role of the CPDI in advancing the scientific foundations of CPD. Its overall role is of encouraging collaboration and establishing leadership in achieving consensus. The committee concluded that research priorities should be set in a collaborative manner and could be performed either by a separate research organization analogous to EPOC or by the CPDI.

Research Areas

CPD activities have not been consistently evaluated. To make a case for investing in CPD, the research enterprise must begin such evaluations. In its evaluation of the literature, the committee identified areas where research is immediately needed. These research areas include evaluation of CPD effectiveness and efficiency methods; best learning methods and lifelong learning; development and validation of measurements and evaluation instruments; impact of CPD on health outcomes; and the effects of planned change initiatives, including regulation. To more rapidly advance the field, efforts in these areas should address what works and why or why not.

The existing CPD literature is often limited by inappropriate choice of methods, research goals, and questions and by hypotheses not built on theories that can grow and develop as they are tested. Without an organized body of knowledge about the effectiveness and efficiency of efforts to impact change, the value of CPD cannot be assessed and health professionals cannot depend on it as a vehicle for improving practices and patient health. Research on the effectiveness of CPD must also align CPD activities with the identified needs and appropriate skills to be learned. For example, research should recognize that lectures may be good for transmitting information, but other methods are needed for deeper learning and performance change. Research is siloed by discipline and, although it may have implications for other disciplines, is often ignored but is critical for developers, users of CPD activities, and policy makers.

Little evidence compares CPD methods, making it difficult to understand how best to enhance professional development. For example, what methods yield the greatest benefit for improved quality of care? In what contexts? How much interactive learning is necessary? How much feedback and simulation are called for? Research should be conducted on the utility of these methods individually and their particular circumstances to determine the best mix to produce changes in health professional performance, thereby improving patient outcomes. This research is necessary to better understand how resources should best be spent and includes explorations of the lifelong learning process.

Strong research requires the development and validation of measurement and evaluation instruments. Current research methods are not necessarily appropriate for addressing the highest-priority research questions; CPD research methods should incorporate methods from the social sciences, in addition to the more traditional clinical sciences. In health services research, qualitative methods in particular are poorly understood and poorly employed, limiting the ability to explain randomized trials and systematic reviews. Some of this limitation may be due to the diversity of researchers and research paradigms, as well as the paucity of opportunities to train those who conduct research about CPD for the health professions.

It is necessary to define and explicitly describe the specific relationships among variables that explain the success or failure of CPD to achieve the desired health outcomes. It is also necessary to associate explicitly the variety of measures useful to assess whether outcomes have been achieved. In this case, the term *health outcomes* includes the individual, systems, and population levels. For the individual clinician, enhanced knowledge and skills must be assessed to ascertain whether he is not only learning the necessary information to maintain and improve competence, but also allowing this information to inform practice. This leads to a second type of outcome—performance measures on clinical outcomes, such as treatment efficacy and disease prevention. On a systems level, data on equitable treatment should be collected to ensure that all subpopulations—including racial and ethnic, gender, age, and community—are receiving the best possible care. Systems outcomes must also be evaluated, such as resource management; cost effectiveness; patient safety; and reduction of overuse, misuse, and underuse of services.

Finally, the effects of planned change (e.g., process mandates, academic detailing), including regulation, should also be explored, as policies regarding CPD are considered. The CPD system should continuously be evaluated to ensure that it meets its goals of improving quality and patient safety.

Many gaps exist in the current literature, highlighting the incomplete nature of the current research system. Research in the above suggested areas and criteria would provide guidance for how to better invest resources and will facilitate future evaluations of CPD. It will also be important to train researchers to use appropriate research methods. To this end, the research workforce needs to be better prepared and provide incentives to develop the research capacity to adequately study the identified research areas.

Innovative methods require testing for effectiveness before being broadly disseminated. Newer, innovative CPD methods should be tested through demonstration programs. For example, learning portfolios can be used across professions to improve the learning process, but the effectiveness of learning portfolios in this capacity must be assessed before investments are made to use them to track the performance of health professionals widely. Demonstration programs can be developed using the research and development structures currently in place.

Recommendation 9: Supporting mobilization of research findings to advance health professional performance, agencies that support demonstration programs, such as the Agency for Healthcare Research and Quality and the Health Resources and Services Administration, should collaborate with the institute.

EVALUATION

Continuing professional development is a complex system involving the collaboration of many stakeholders. To ensure that the system and the Continuing Professional Development Institute are functioning properly and progress is being made toward better health professional development, evaluation must be performed continually that is supported by data. Initially, evaluation ought to occur at four levels: individual health professionals, stakeholder organizations, the CPDI, and the overall CPD system. The Council on Data Collection and Dissemination would be helpful in developing strategies for collecting this data. Accountability at each level is critical for success but will require different evaluation metrics. Other levels of evaluation, for example teams and health care systems, ought to be considered upon greater ability to measure effectiveness.

Advances or declines in health professional competence are integral to determining how effective the system is. Measures should be developed to evaluate improvement and maintenance of individual health professionals' competence that might align with higher levels of outcomes that pertain to individual practitioners. Such evaluations could also be reported in ways similar to public reporting of performance measures, holding practitioners responsible for their own learning. It will be important to evaluate the learning methods, context, and outcomes together to further implementation and dissemination.

Separate evaluations are also needed of stakeholders, allowing for the specific diagnosis of particular parts of the CPD system, in their given contexts. This includes researchers, CPD providers, regulatory bodies, employers, and payers. These entities would be assessed based on individually identified measures, offering health professionals support in providing cost-effective, conflict-free learning activities to enhance quality care. The CPDI would not necessarily perform the evaluations but would instead hold others accountable for assessing the effectiveness of the components of the CPD system in a timely manner.

The CPDI itself should also be assessed periodically by an external evaluator. Each of its four main areas should have specific goals and metrics for evaluation. The CPDI should also be held accountable to measures of its relationships with stakeholders, operation of councils and ad hoc committees, and accomplishment of the research agenda.

Arguably the most important but most difficult level of evaluation is that of the overall system of CPD. The CPDI should be held accountable by the public for its activities and stewardship of the CPD system, through provision of periodic reports to the Secretary. Reports about the state of CPD would begin after 2-5 years to allow for the start of the CPDI. This would be analogous to Medicare Payment Advisory Commission (MedPAC) reports, which advise the public on the state of Medicare payments and the Congress on how to continuously improve the payment system.

Recommendation 10: The Continuing Professional Development Institute should report annually to its public and private stakeholders and should hold a national symposium on the performance and progress of professional development education and its role in enhancing quality and patient safety.

HOW WILL WE KNOW WHEN WE GET THERE?

It will be necessary for the CPDI to evaluate its progress continuously so that it can adjust its approaches to enhance health professionals' learning. It will also be necessary to know when the system has achieved its end goals of serving health care professionals, their employers, and payers. An ideal system should also foster functional team-based care, be learner-driven, decrease costs, and improve health outcomes.

Interim measures toward these goals will need to be developed to continuously evaluate the CPD system. For example, measures to evaluate the CPD system and the micro-, meso-, and macrosystems could be used to hold the overall system accountable. Tracking advances in the literature and regulatory changes are relatively simple ways to gauge progress and should be considered. Efforts to collect data at the levels of individual professionals, organizations, and professions to determine whether these goals have been successfully achieved should be led by the Council on Data Collection and Dissemination. To this end, the CPDI should foster a learning system, constantly building on its own successes and failures.

CONSEQUENCES OF INACTION

A well-educated workforce is necessary for improving health care. But despite the long period of professional training and the nature of today's information-rich health care environment, it remains unclear whether health professionals are effectively and efficiently learning in ways that maintain minimum levels of competence and help improve performance. During the past 30 years, research shows limited effects of continuing education in applied learning opportunities. This must change toward a system that more definitively asserts the value and effectiveness of learning in health care.

The status quo is unacceptable; poor quality of care continues to threaten patient safety, further fragment the system, and potentially increase waste. Inaction would signify society's unwillingness to support health professional development to systematically improve quality and patient safety in a timely manner. The root of the problem lies with the culture and environment in which health professionals practice, inhibiting them from providing the best possible care.

Although difficult, change is possible and needs to overcome the many challenges facing CPD. Reform is needed to provide health professionals with the capacity to perform to their highest potential. The CPD system needs to be coordinated and harmonized, but cannot and will not be without a central convener. With cooperation and central coordination, clinicians can continuously and systemically improve, raising their levels of knowledge and competence in the care of patients by functional teams. Action must result in the advances needed to assure the public of the health care workforce's ability to provide high quality, safe care.

REFERENCES

ABMS (American Board of Medical Specialties). 2009. *ABMS maintenance of certification.* http://abms.org/Maintenance_of_Certification/ABMS_MOC.aspx (accessed April 23, 2009).

ACCME (Accreditation Council on Continuing Medical Education). 2009. *Joint accreditation for the provider of continuing education for the healthcare team.* http://www.accme.org/index.cfm/fa/news.detail/News/.cfm/news_id/a71d122c-0a81-45c1-ad90-b71af47739c3.cfm (accessed April 15, 2009).

EPOC (Effective Practice and Organisation of Care). 2009. *Priority topics.* http://epocoslo.cochrane.org/en/publications.html (accessed April 24, 2009).

FSMB (Federation of State Medical Boards). 2008. *Special Committee on Maintenance of Licensure draft report on maintenance of licensure.* http://www.fsmb.org/pdf/Special_Committee_MOL_Draft_Report_February2008.pdf (accessed July 30, 2009).

HRSA (Health Resources and Services Administration). 2005. *Strategic plan FY 2005-2010: Goal #2—Improve health outcomes.* Rockville, MD: U.S. Department of Health and Human Services, HRSA.

———. 2009. *About HRSA.* http://www.hrsa.gov/about/default.htm (accessed April 17, 2009).

IOM (Institute of Medicine). 2003. *Health professions education: A bridge to quality.* Washington, DC: The National Academies Press.

Nelson, E. C., P. B. Batalden, and M. M. Godfrey, eds. 2007. *Quality by design: A clinical microsystems approach.* 1st ed. San Francisco, CA: Jossey-Bass.

NPP (National Priorities Partnership). 2008. *National priorities and goals: Executive summary.* Washington, DC: National Quality Forum.

Slutsky, J., D. Atkins, and S. Chang. 2008. Comparing medical interventions: AHRQ and the effective health care program. In *Methods guide for comparative effectiveness reviews.* Edited by the Agency for Healthcare Research and Quality. Rockville, MD.

Whitlock, E. P., S. A. Lopez, S. Chang, M. Helfand, M. Eder, and N. Floyd. 2009. Identifying, selecting, and refining topics. In *Methods guide for comparative effectiveness reviews.* Edited by the Agency for Healthcare Research and Quality. Rockville, MD.

Appendix A

Literature Review Tables

Evidence on the effectiveness of continuing education (CE) and CE methods was identified through a literature review. Although nonexhaustive, the review included a comprehensive search of the Research and Development Resource Base (RDRB), a bibliographic database of more than 18,000 articles from fields including CE, knowledge translation, interprofessional literature, and faculty development. Articles in the RDRB are culled from Medline, the Cumulative Index to Nursing and Allied Health Literature (CINAHL), Excerpta Medica Database (EMBASE), Education Resources Information Center (ERIC), Sociological Abstracts, PsychoInfo, Library Information and Science Abstracts (LISA), and business databases, as well as automatic retrieval of articles from journals dedicated to medical education (e.g., *Journal of Continuing Education in the Health Professions, Medical Education, Studies in Continuing Education*).

The RDRB was searched using keywords,[1] and the results of the searches were culled by two independent reviewers using an iterative approach. Studies collected were from 1989 to April 2009.

---

[1] Keywords used to search the RDRB included "patient participation," "patient initiated," "patient mediated," "physician prompt," "audit," "feedback," "checklist," "checklists," "protocol," "protocols," "reminder," "reminders," "academic detailing," "simulation," "simulations," "lifelong learning," "experiential," "self-directed," "reflection," "problem based," "model," and "modeling." These keywords were used alone or in combination.

Abstracts of search results were reviewed to eliminate articles that clearly did not pertain to CE methods, cost-effectiveness, or educational theory and to categorize the studies as informative, equivocal, or not informative of CE effectiveness. A wide range of designs were classified as informative, including randomized controlled trials, prospective cohort studies, observational studies, and studies with pre- and post-intervention assessment methodologies. Quantitative and qualitative approaches were included, and inclusion was not limited to studies with positive results. The most common reasons articles were classified as not informative were absence of a trial design, small sample size, and high likelihood of confounding factors in the design that could affect outcomes. The two reviewers independently classified abstracts and full texts of the articles and then compared their classification results. Interreviewer reliability was greater than 80 percent, and discrepancies were resolved by a consensus process. A third reviewer verified the results classified as informative or equivocal in a final round of detailed assessment of the study design, populations, intervention, type of outcome, and conclusions for each article. Systematic reviews and meta-analyses are included in Table A-1; studies and articles are included in Table A-2.

Table A-1 begins on the next page.

TABLE A-1 Summary of Systematic Reviews on Effectiveness of CE Methods

Reference	Purpose	Number of Studies, Inclusion Criteria, and Databases Searched
Reflection		
Ruth-Sahd, L. A. 2003. Reflective practice: A critical analysis of data-based studies and implications for nursing education. *Journal of Nursing Education* 42(11):488-497.	* Identify common themes that emerge from data-based studies * Identify implications for reflective practice in the field of nursing education	**Sample:** 20 articles, 12 doctoral dissertations, and 6 books **Inclusion criteria:** Delineated methodology section; emphasis on reflective practice in an education setting; publication between 1992 and 2002; English language **Databases:** CINAHL, Dissertation Abstracts International, ERIC, PsychInfo
Simulation		
Issenberg, S. B., W. C. McGaghie, E. R. Petrusa, D. L. Gordon, and R. J. Scalese. 2005. Features and uses of high-fidelity medical simulations that lead to effective learning: A BEME systematic review. *Medical Teacher* 27:10-28.	Determine the features and uses of high-fidelity medical simulators that lead to the most effective learning (high-fidelity simulators are models, mannequins, or virtual packages that utilize realistic materials and equipment and incorporate feedback, computerized control, or other advanced technology)	**Sample:** 109 articles **Inclusion criteria:** Empirical study; use of a simulator as an education assessment or intervention; learner outcomes measured quantitatively; experimental or quasi-experimental design **Databases:** ERIC, Medline, PsychInfo, Web of Science, Timelit

Main Results	Limitations
* Conditions necessary for reflection to be successful: • Active motivation • Safe learning environments • Time availability * Students require guidance about how to practice reflection	* No research on how unconscious knowledge is affected by reflective practice * Lack of hypothesis testing in reviewed studies
High fidelity simulators facilitate learning under certain conditions: • Repetitive practice • Used in conjunction with multiple learning strategies • Variety of clinical conditions captured • Controlled environment where errors can be made and corrected • Individualized learning where participants are actively involved	Heterogeneity of research designs, educational interventions, outcome measures, and time frame precluded data synthesis using meta-analysis

continued

TABLE A-1 Continued

Reference	Purpose	Number of Studies, Inclusion Criteria, and Databases Searched
Sutherland, L. M., P. F. Middleton, A. Anthony, J. Hamdorf, P. Cregan, D. Scott, and G. J. Maddern. 2006. Surgical simulation: A systematic review. *Annals of Surgery* 243(3):291-300.	Evaluate the effectiveness of surgical simulation compared with other methods of surgical training	**Sample:** 30 trials with 760 participants **Inclusion criteria:** Randomized controlled trial; assessing surgical simulation; measures of surgical task performance **Databases:** Medline, EMBASE, Cochrane Library, PsycINFO, CINAHL, Science Citation Index

Reminders

Balas, E. A., S. M. Austin, J. A. Mitchell, B. G. Ewigman, K. D. Bopp, and G. D. Brown. 1996. The clinical value of computerized information services. A review of 98 randomized clinical trials. *Archives of Family Medicine* 5(5):271-278.	Determine the clinical settings, types of interventions, and effects of studies in randomized clinical trials addressing the efficacy of clinical information systems	**Sample:** 98 articles reporting on 100 trials **Inclusion criteria:** Randomized controlled trial (RCT); computerized information intervention in the experimental group; effect measured on the process or outcome of care **Databases:** Medline
Shea, S., W. DuMouchel, and L. Bahamonde. 1996. A meta-analysis of 16 randomized controlled trials to evaluate computer-based clinical reminder systems for preventive care in the ambulatory setting. *Journal of the American Medical Informatics Association* 3(6):399-409.	Assess the overall effectiveness of computer-based reminder systems in ambulatory settings directed at preventive care	**Sample:** 16 trials **Inclusion criteria:** Randomized controlled trial; computer-based reminder; control group received no intervention **Databases:** Medline, Nursing and Allied Health database, Health Planning and Administration database

Main Results	Limitations
Computer simulation generally showed better results than no training at all but was not superior to standard training (e.g., surgical drills) or video simulation	Insufficient evidence to evaluate types of simulation because outcomes were often not comparable across studies
Patient and physician reminders, computerized treatment planners, and interactive patient education can make a significant difference in managing care ($P < 0.05$)	Many trials evaluate the effect of information services on care processes as opposed to patient outcomes
* Computer reminders improved preventive practices for vaccinations, breast cancer screening, colorectal cancer screening, and cardiovascular screening * Computerized reminders did not improve preventive practices for cervical cancer screening	Heterogeneity in study designs and the ways in which results were presented

continued

TABLE A-1 Continued

Reference	Purpose	Number of Studies, Inclusion Criteria, and Databases Searched
Audit and Feedback		
Jamtvedt, G., J. M. Young, D. T. Kristoffersen, M. A. O'Brien, and A. D. Oxman. 2006. Does telling people what they have been doing change what they do? A systematic review of the effects of audit and feedback. *Quality & Safety in Health Care* 15(6):433-436.	Review the effects of audit and feedback on improving professional practice	**Sample:** 118 trials **Inclusion criteria:** Randomized controlled trials; utilized audit and feedback; objective measures of provider performance **Databases:** Cochrane Library
Multifaceted Interventions and Reviews of Multiple Methods		
Cheraghi-Sohi, S., and P. Bower. 2008. Can the feedback of patient assessments, brief training, or their combination, improve the interpersonal skills of primary care physicians? A systematic review. *BMC Health Services Research* 8.	* Review the efficacy of patient feedback on the interpersonal care skills of primary care physicians * Review the efficacy of brief training (up to one working week in length) focused on the improvement of interpersonal care	**Sample:** 9 studies **Inclusion criteria:** Randomized controlled trials; published in English; based on primary care practitioners and their patients; utilized patient feedback or brief training or a combination of these methods; outcome measure was a patient-based assessment in change **Databases:** CENTRAL, Medline, EMBASE

Main Results	Limitations
* Effects of audit and feedback on improving professional practice are generally small to moderate * Effects of audit and feedback are likely to be larger when baseline adherence to recommended practice is low and audit and feedback are delivered more frequently and over longer periods of time	* Lack of a process evaluation embedded in trials * Few studies compare audit and feedback to other interventions
Brief training as currently delivered is not effective	* Limited evidence on the effects of patient-based feedback for changes in primary care physician behavior * Evidence is not definitive due to the small number of trials * Variation in training methods and goals * Lack of theory linking feedback to behavior change

continued

TABLE A-1 Continued

Reference	Purpose	Number of Studies, Inclusion Criteria, and Databases Searched
Davis, D., M. A. O'Brien, N. Freemantle, F. M. Wolf, P. Mazmanian, and A. Taylor-Vaisey. 1999. Impact of formal continuing medical education: Do conferences, workshops, rounds, and other traditional continuing education activities change physician behavior or health care outcomes? *JAMA* 282(9):867-874.	Review, collate, and interpret the effect of formal continuing medical education (CME) interventions on physician performance and health care outcomes	**Sample:** 14 studies **Inclusion criteria:** Randomized controlled trial of formal didactic and/or interactive CME; >50% physicians **Databases:** RDRB, Cochrane Library, Medline
Forsetlund, L., A. Bjørndal, A. Rashidian, G. Jamtvedt, M. A. O'Brien, F. Wolf, D. Davis, J. Odgaard-Jensen, and A. D. Oxman. 2009. Continuing education meetings and workshops: Effects on professional practice and health care outcomes. *Cochrane Database Systematic Reviews* (2):CD003030.	To assess the effects of educational meetings on professional practice and health care outcomes	**Sample:** 81 trials involving more than 11,000 health professionals **Inclusion criteria:** Randomized controlled trial of educational meetings that reported an objective measure of professional practice or health care outcomes **Databases:** Cochrane Library
Grimshaw, J., L. Shirran, R. Thomas, G. Mowatt, C. Fraser, L. Bero, R. Grilli, E. Harvey, A. Oxman, and M. A. O'Brien. 2001. Changing provider behavior: An overview of systematic reviews of interventions. *Medical Care* 39(8 Suppl 2):II2-II45.	Identify, appraise, and synthesize systematic reviews of professional education or quality assurance interventions to improve quality of care	**Sample:** 41 reviews **Inclusion criteria:** Interventions targeted at health professionals; reported measures of professional performance and/or patient outcomes; study design included explicit selection criteria **Databases:** Medline, Healthstar, Cochrane Library

Main Results	Limitations
* Interactive CME sessions that enhance participant activity and provide the opportunity to practice skills can effect change in professional practice and, on occasion, health outcomes * Didactic sessions did not appear to be effective in changing physician performance	* Limited number of randomized controlled trials and settings limits generalizability of findings * The comparability of CME interventions is debatable due to the lack of comparability of reviewed interventions
* Educational meetings alone are not likely to be effective for changing behaviors * The effect of educational meetings combined with other interventions is most likely to be small and similar to other types of CE, such as audit and feedback, and educational outreach visits	* Heterogeneity in study designs and the ways in which results were presented * Observed differences in changing behaviors cannot be explained with confidence
* Passive approaches generally ineffective * Active approaches effective under some circumstances * Multifaceted interventions more likely to be effective than interventions with one method	Lack of agreement within the research community on a theoretical or empirical framework for classifying interventions

continued

TABLE A-1 Continued

Reference	Purpose	Number of Studies, Inclusion Criteria, and Databases Searched
Gross, P. A., and D. Pujat. 2001. Implementing practice guidelines for appropriate antimicrobial usage: A systematic review. *Medical Care* 39(8 Suppl 2):II55-II69.	* Conduct a systematic review of guideline implementation studies for improving appropriate use of antimicrobial agents * Determine which implementation methods appear to improve the outcome of appropriate antimicrobial use	**Sample:** 40 studies **Inclusion criteria:** Comparative study; quantitative data; English language; between 1966 and 2000 **Databases:** Medline
Lam-Antoniades, M., S. Ratnapalan, and G. Tait. 2009. Electronic continuing education in the health professions: An update on evidence from RCTs. *Journal of Continuing Education in the Health Professions* 29:44-51.	Update evidence from RCTs assessing the effectiveness of electronic CE (e-CE)	**Sample:** 15 studies **Inclusion criteria:** Evaluated a CE intervention for any group of health professionals; intervention included a computer interface (CD-ROM or Internet); randomized controlled trial; published between 2004 and 2007 **Databases:** Medline, EMBASE, CINAHL
Marinopoulos, S. S., T. Dorman, N. Ratanawongsa, L. M. Wilson, B. H. Ashar, J. L. Magaziner, R. G. Miller, P. A. Thomas, G. P. Prokopowicz, R. Qayyum, and E. B. Bass. 2007. *Effectiveness of continuing medical education.* Evidence report/technology assessment no. 149. AHRQ Publication No. 07-E006. Rockville, MD: Agency for Healthcare Research and Quality.	Synthesize evidence regarding the effectiveness of CME and differing instructional designs in terms of knowledge, attitudes, skills, practice behavior, and clinical practice outcomes	**Sample:** 136 articles and 9 systematic reviews **Inclusion criteria:** Reporting on the effects of CME or simulation; written in English; contained original human data; included at least 15 fully trained physicians; evaluated an educational activity; published between 1981 and 2006; conducted in the United States or Canada; included data from a comparison group **Databases:** Medline, EMBASE, Cochrane Library, PsycINFO, ERIC

Main Results	Limitations
* Multifaceted implementation methods most successful * Individual implementation methods determined to be useful: • Academic detailing • Feedback from nurses, pharmacists, or physicians • Local adoption of a guideline • Small-group interactive sessions • Computer-assisted care	* Multimethod approaches make it difficult to determine which method(s) were critical for appropriate antimicrobial use * Findings may not be generalizable because study conditions vary
* Positive effects of e-CE on knowledge sustained up to 12 months * Positive effects of e-CE on practice sustained up to 5 months * e-CE interventions that only included text via reading passages of limited effectiveness in changing knowledge or practice	None of the studies attempted to identify which components of a multifaceted intervention were responsible for effects
* CME effective in achieving and maintaining knowledge, attitudes, skills, practice behavior, and clinical practice outcomes * Live media more effective than print; multimedia more effective than single-media interventions; multiple exposures more effective than a single exposure	* Firm conclusions not possible because of overall low quality of the literature * Heterogeneity in study designs and the ways in which results were presented * Limited evidence on reliability and validity of the tools used to assess CME effectiveness

continued

TABLE A-1 Continued

Reference	Purpose	Number of Studies, Inclusion Criteria, and Databases Searched
Mansouri, M., and J. Lockyer. 2007. A meta-analysis of continuing medical education effectiveness. *Journal of Continuing Education in the Health Professions* 27:6-15.	Examine the effect of moderator variables on physician knowledge, performance, and patient outcomes	**Sample:** 31 studies **Inclusion criteria:** Randomized controlled trial or before-and-after experimental design; participants were practicing physicians; focus on at least 1 of the 3 identified outcomes (physician knowledge, physician performance, patient outcome); adequate description of the intervention; quantitative analyses **Databases:** Medline, ERIC
O'Brien, M. A., N. Freemantle, A. D. Oxman, F. Wolf, D. A. Davis, and J. Herrin. 2001. Continuing education meetings and workshops: Effects on professional practice and health care outcomes. *Cochrane Database of Systematic Reviews (Online)* (2).	Assess the effects of educational meetings on professional practice and health care outcomes	**Sample:** 32 studies **Inclusion criteria:** Randomized trials or quasi-experimental studies; effect of lectures, workshops, and/or courses on clinical practice or health care outcomes **Databases:** Cochrane Library, Medline, RDRB
Prior, M., M. Guerin, and K. Grimmer-Somers. 2008. The effectiveness of clinical guideline implementation strategies—A synthesis of systematic review findings. *Journal of Evaluation in Clinical Practice* 14(5):888-897.	Synthesize evidence of effectiveness of clinical guideline implementation strategies in terms of improved clinical processes and improved cost-benefit ratios	**Sample:** 33 systematic reviews that included 714 primary studies **Inclusion criteria:** Generic implementation strategies; comparison study; measured clinical practice change and/or compliance; published between 1987 and 2007; English language **Databases:** Medline, Amed, CINAHL, Academic Search Elite, Cochrane Library

Main Results	Limitations
* Larger effect size when the interventions are interactive ($r = 0.33$ [0.33]) and use multiple methods ($r = 0.33$ [0.26]) * Larger effect size for longer interventions ($r = 0.33$) and multiple interventions over time ($r = 0.36$) * Smaller effect size for programs with multiple professions ($r = -0.18$) and a greater number of participants ($r = -0.13$)	Studies did not always provide • Descriptive information about the participants or the intervention • Statistical information using accepted standards for reporting • Numeric data • Validity and reliability data • Data about the period of time between the intervention and the measurement of performance
* Interactive workshops can result in changes in professional practice * Didactic sessions alone unlikely to change professional practice	* Study design generally poorly reported, making it difficult to judge the degree to which results may be biased * Substantial variation in the complexity of targeted behaviors, baseline compliance, and the characteristics of interventions * Heterogeneity in study designs and the ways in which results were presented
* Implementation strategies where there was strong evidence of guideline compliance included • Multifaceted interventions • Interactive education • Clinical reminder systems * Didactic education and passive dissemination strategies (e.g., conferences, websites) ineffective	* Implementation strategies varied and rarely comparable * Cost-effectiveness analyses rare

continued

TABLE A-1 Continued

Reference	Purpose	Number of Studies, Inclusion Criteria, and Databases Searched
Robertson, M. A., K. E. Umble, and R. M. Cervero. 2003. Impact studies in continuing education for health professions: Update. *Journal of Continuing Education in the Health Professions* 23:146-156.	* Determine if CE is effective and for what outcomes * Determine what kinds of CE are effective	**Sample:** 15 syntheses **Inclusion criteria:** Primary CE study; professionals' performance and/or patient health outcomes considered; published since 1993 **Databases:** RDRB, Medline, ERIC, Digital Dissertation Abstracts
Steinman, M. A., S. R. Ranji, K. G. Shojania, and R. Gonzales. 2006. Improving antibiotic selection: A systematic review and quantitative analysis of quality improvement strategies. *Medical Care* 44(7):617-628.	Assess which interventions are most effective at improving the prescribing of recommended antibiotics for acute outpatient infections	**Sample:** 26 studies reporting on 33 trials **Inclusion criteria:** Clinical trial; reports on antibiotic selection in acute outpatient infections; randomized trials, controlled before-and-after and interrupted time-series designs with at least 3 data points; English language **Databases:** Cochrane Library, Medline
Tian, J., N. L. Atkinson, B. Portnoy, and R. S. Gold. 2007. A systematic review of evaluation in formal continuing medical education. *Journal of Continuing Education in the Health Professions* 27:16-27.	Improve CME evaluation study design by determining • Effects of using randomization strategies on outcome measurement • Reliability and validity of measurement • Follow-up period recommendations	**Sample:** 32 studies **Inclusion criteria:** Randomized controlled trial or quasi-experimental trial; published between 1993 and 1999; primary studies; >50% physicians; CME intervention was didactic, interactive, or both **Databases:** Medline, EBSCOhost

Main Results	Limitations
* CE can improve knowledge, skills, attitudes, behavior, and patient health outcomes * Effective CE is ongoing, interactive, contextually relevant, and based on needs assessment	* Few primary studies addressed the impact of CE on patient health outcomes (and instead measured patient satisfaction) * Focus on how CE affects individuals as opposed to teams or organizations
Multidimensional interventions using audit and feedback less effective than interventions using clinician education alone	* Sample size too small to conduct detailed analysis of all potential confounders and effect modifiers * Heterogeneity in study designs and the ways in which results were presented
* Valid and reliable questionnaire addressing variables necessary to allow comparison of effectiveness across interventions * Minimum 1-year post-intervention period necessary to investigate sustainability of outcomes	Variation across study designs prevents comparing the effectiveness of CME programs

continued

TABLE A-1 Continued

Reference	Purpose	Number of Studies, Inclusion Criteria, and Databases Searched
Tu, K., and D. A. Davis. 2002. Can we alter physician behavior by educational methods? Lessons learned from studies of the management and follow-up of hypertension. *Journal of Continuing Education in the Health Professions* 22(1):11-22.	Review the literature on the effectiveness of physician educational interventions in the management and follow-up of hypertension	**Sample:** 12 studies **Inclusion criteria:** Use of replicable educational interventions; >50% physician involvement; objective measures of physician behavior change or patient outcomes; dropout rate of <30%; outcomes assessed for >30 days **Databases:** PubMed, RDRB
Wensing, M., H. Wollersheim, and R. Grol. 2006. Organizational interventions to implement improvements in patient care: A structured review of reviews. *Implementation Science* 1(1).	Provide an overview of the research evidence on the effects of organizational strategies to implement improvements in patient care	**Sample:** 36 reviews **Inclusion Criteria:** Evaluated organizational strategies; published in 1995 or later; rigorous evaluations (e.g., randomized trials, interrupted time-series, controlled before-and-after, and prospective comparative observational studies) **Databases:** PubMed, Cochrane Library

Main Results	Limitations
* Studies included 7 different educational interventions: reminders, formal CME, computerized decision support, printed materials, academic detailing, continuous quality improvement, and prompts	* Relatively small number of trials in each of the types of interventions * Randomized trials using quantitative outcomes do not capture processes and dimensions of learning
* Professional performance was generally improved by revision of professional roles and utilization of computer systems for knowledge management * Multidisciplinary teams, integrated care services, and computer systems generally improved patient outcomes	Heterogeneity in study designs and the ways in which results were presented

TABLE A-2 Literature Review on the Effectiveness of CE Methods

Reference	Study Purpose	Sample, Method, Outcome Measures, and Duration
Experiential and Self-Directed Learning		
East, D., and K. Jacoby. 2005. The effect of a nursing staff education program on compliance with central line care policy in the cardiac intensive care unit. *Pediatric Nursing* 31(3):182-184.	Demonstrate the effectiveness of a self-study education module on nurse compliance with central line care policy	**Sample:** 20 registered nurses (RNs) in a 12-bed pediatric cardiovascular intensive care unit **Method:** Quasi-experimental cohort study with pre- and post-test design **Outcome measures:** Compliance with 10 central line policies; intravenous (IV) line audit tool used to collect data on 47 patients pre- and post-intervention **Duration:** 7 months
Hewson, M. G., H. L. Copeland, E. Mascha, S. Arrigain, E. Topol, and J. E. Fox. 2006. Integrative medicine: Implementation and evaluation of a professional development program using experiential learning and conceptual change teaching approaches. *Patient Education & Counseling* 62(1):5-12.	Raise physicians' awareness of, and initiate attitudinal changes toward, integrative medicine through a professional development program involving experiential learning	**Sample:** 48 cardiologists at an academic medical center **Method:** Randomized controlled trial • Experimental group: participation in intervention • Control group: no intervention **Outcome measure:** Self-reported knowledge, attitudes, likelihood of changing practice, and satisfaction **Duration:** 8 hours

Description of Educational Method	Findings
Self-study module included a fact sheet and poster outlining proper care	Self-study had a statistically significant impact on staff compliance with central line policy ($p < 0.001$, 95% CI)
Professional development session in which participants participated in integrative medicine modalities (e.g., yoga, Reiki)	* Participant group had significant positive changes in their conceptions about and attitudes to complementary and alternative medicine after the program * Physicians significantly increased their willingness to integrate CAM into their practice

continued

TABLE A-2 Continued

Reference	Study Purpose	Sample, Method, Outcome Measures, and Duration
Karner, K. J., D. C. Rheinheimer, A. M. DeLisi, and C. Due. 1998. The impact of a hospital-wide experiential learning educational program on staff's knowledge and misconceptions about aging. *Journal of Continuing Education in Nursing* 29(3):100-104.	Examine the impact on the knowledge and attitudes of hospital personnel of their participation in an experiential learning program to increase knowledge about aging	**Sample:** 95 hospital employees (administrative, nursing, social work, occupational therapy, physical therapy, dietary, maintenance, and pastoral care) **Method:** Cohort study with pre- and post-test design **Outcome measures:** Knowledge gains as evidenced by improvement on a 25-question exam about the feelings of older people; bias as determined by responses on the exam **Duration:** 2 hours
Love, B., C. McAdams, D. M. Patton, E. J. Rankin, and J. Roberts. 1989. Teaching psychomotor skills in nursing: A randomized control trial. *Journal of Advanced Nursing* 14(11):970-975.	Compare the effectiveness of teaching psychomotor skills in a structured laboratory setting with self-directed, self-taught modules	**Sample:** 77 second-year students in a baccalaureate nursing program in Ontario, Canada **Method:** Randomized controlled trial • Experimental group: clinical laboratory training • Control group: self-directed learning **Outcome measure:** Achievement as measured by the Objective Structured Clinical Examination (OSCE) **Duration:** One clinical term

Description of Educational Method	Findings
One-hour role-play game designed for participants to experience and then reflect on their feelings toward older people	* Significant increase in scores between pre-test and post-test ($F = 64.08$, $p < 0.0001$) * Negative bias scores decreased significantly from pre- to post-test ($F = 23.86$, $p < 0.0001$)
* Packets containing information on specific skills, definitions, resources, problem-solving scenarios were distributed * Learners watched expert clinicians	No difference between psychomotor skill performance of students who learned in a self-directed manner and those taught in a structured clinical laboratory

continued

TABLE A-2 Continued

Reference	Study Purpose	Sample, Method, Outcome Measures, and Duration
Russell, J. M. 1990. Relationships among preference for educational structure, self-directed learning, instructional methods, and achievement. *Journal of Professional Nursing* 6(2):86-93.	Analyze nurses' preference for educational structure, self-directed learning, instructional method, and achievement on a written exam	**Sample:** 40 RNs in 8 community hospitals **Method:** Randomized controlled trial • Experimental group: self-directed learning • Control group: lecture **Outcome measures:** Scores on a 50-item post-test; scores on the Self-Directed Learning Readiness Scale **Duration:** 1 week
Suggs, P. K., M. B. Mittelmark, R. Krissak, K. Oles, C. Lane, Jr., and B. Richards. 1998. Efficacy of a self-instruction package when compared with a traditional continuing education offering for nurses. *Journal of Continuing Education in the Health Professions* 18(4):220-226.	Determine whether a multimedia, self-instructional education package can provide similar learning results as received from a conventional CE conference	**Sample:** 63 RNs and licensed practical nurses (LPNs) in 2 rural regions in North and South Carolina **Method:** Ecologic study • Experimental group: self-instructed course • Control group: traditional CE course **Outcome measure:** Knowledge gains evaluated by a pre- and post-multiple-choice test **Duration:** NA

Reflection

Reference	Study Purpose	Sample, Method, Outcome Measures, and Duration
Forneris, S. G., and C. Peden-McAlpine. 2007. Evaluation of a reflective learning intervention to improve critical thinking in novice nurses. *Journal of Advanced Nursing* 57(4):410-421.	Determine if a reflective contextual learning intervention would improve novice nurses' critical thinking skills during their first 6 months of practice	**Sample:** 6 novice nurse-nurse preceptor dyads at an urban acute care facility **Method:** Qualitative case study **Outcome measures:** Self-reported anxiety, influence of power, use of questioning, use of sequential thinking, use of contextual thinking **Duration:** 6 months

Description of Educational Method	Findings
Self-directed group received reading materials, audio tapes, self-evaluation tests, case study analyses, and an instruction session for clarification	* No significant relationships found between exam scores and self-directed learning readiness ($p = 0.24$) * No participant in the self-directed group chose to participate in an instructor clarification session
* 5-hour CE workshop delivered by a pharmacist * Self-paced 6- to 10-hour instructional education package with videotapes, a workbook with case histories, and a textbook	* Both control and experimental groups had statistically significant improvement ($t = 4.86$, $p < 0.0001$ and $t = -2.54$, $p < 0.18$, respectively) * Knowledge gains were not significantly higher for the control group
* Narrative journals * Daily coaching to help incorporate critical thinking into practice * Leader-facilitated discussion groups	* Lack of trust in one's knowledge base influenced how an individual used critical thinking * Thinking out loud allowed nurses to verbalize sources of knowledge and plan actions * Contextual learning assisted in the development of critical thinking * Sustainability of critical thinking skills post-intervention unknown

continued

TABLE A-2 Continued

Reference	Study Purpose	Sample, Method, Outcome Measures, and Duration
Mathers, N. J., M. C. Challis, A. C. Howe, and N. J. Field. 1999. Portfolios in continuing medical education—Effective and efficient? *Medical Education* 33(7):521-530.	Evaluate the effectiveness and efficiency of portfolios for the continuing professional development of general practitioners (GPs)	**Sample:** 32 general practitioners in Sheffield, UK **Method:** Qualitative cohort study comparing traditional CME activities and portfolio-based learning **Outcome measures:** Presence of defined learning objectives; hours of participation in CME activity **Duration:** 12 months
Ranson, S. L., J. Boothby, P. E. Mazmanian, and A. Alvanzo. 2007. Use of personal digital assistants (PDAs) in reflection on learning and practice. *Journal of Continuing Education in the Health Professions* 27:227-233.	Describe the use of (1) personal digital assistants (PDAs) in patient care and (2) a PDA version of a learning portfolio intended to encourage documentation of reflection on practice and medical education	**Sample:** 10 physicians **Method:** Case study **Outcome measures:** PDA usage data; written comments in learning portfolios; self-reported PDA use information **Duration:** 6 months

Academic Detailing

Doyne, E. O., M. P. Alfaro, R. M. Siegel, H. D. Atherton, P. J. Schoettker, J. Bernier, and U. R. Kotagal. 2004. A randomized controlled trial to change antibiotic prescribing patterns in a community. *Archives of Pediatrics and Adolescent Medicine* 158(6):577-583.	Examine the effects of academic detailing on community pediatricians' prescription of antibiotics for children	**Sample:** 12 pediatric practice groups in the greater Cincinnati area **Method:** Cluster randomized controlled trial • Experimental group: report cards and academic detailing visits • Control group: report cards only **Outcome measure:** Antibiotic prescription rate pre- and post-academic detailing **Duration:** 24 months

Description of Educational Method	Findings
3 small-group sessions with a CME tutor to use a portfolio-based learning route to • Identify individual educational needs • Develop strategies to meet these needs • Use reflection to modify objectives	Portfolio learners developed individual learning objectives and had flexibility in methods and timing
Physicians received a PDA preloaded with learning portfolio software and were individually trained in its use	* Use of the PDA associated with the value of information for making clinical decisions * Use of the learning portfolio prompted physicians to reflect on changes in clinical practice
* Each group practice in the experimental group identified 1 leader to present academic detailing sessions to the practice on a monthly basis * Quarterly report cards detailing antibiotic-prescribing data from each practice	* Academic detailing no more effective in reducing antibiotic use than the practice-specific report cards * Antibiotic prescription rate decreased to 0.82 of the baseline rate for the experimental group (95% CI: 0.71-0.95) and to 0.86 of the baseline for the control group (95% CI: 0.77-0.95)

continued

TABLE A-2 Continued

Reference	Study Purpose	Sample, Method, Outcome Measures, and Duration
Goldberg, H. I., E. H. Wagner, S. D. Fihn, D. P. Martin, C. R. Horowitz, D. B. Christensen, A. D. Cheadle, P. Diehr, and G. Simon. 1998. A randomized controlled trial of CQI teams and academic detailing: Can they alter compliance with guidelines? *Joint Commission Journal on Quality Improvement* 24(3):130-142.	Determine the effectiveness of academic detailing techniques and continuous quality improvement teams in increasing compliance with national guidelines for the care of hypertension and depression	**Sample:** 15 small group practices at 4 Seattle primary care clinics **Method:** Randomized controlled trial • Experimental groups: academic detailing; academic detailing and continuous quality improvement (CQI) • Control group: usual care **Outcome measures:** Changes in hypertension prescribing; changes in blood pressure control; changes in depression recognition; changes in use of older tricyclics; changes in scores on the Hopkins Symptom Checklist depression scale **Duration:** 29 months
Goldstein, M. G., R. Niaura, C. Willey, A. Kazura, W. Rakowski, J. DePue, and E. Park. 2003. An academic detailing intervention to disseminate physician-delivered smoking cessation counseling: Smoking cessation outcomes of the Physicians Counseling Smokers Project. *Preventive Medicine* 36(2):185-196.	Determine the effect of a community-based academic detailing intervention on the quit rates of a population-based sample of smokers	**Sample:** 259 primary care physicians and 4,295 adult smokers in Rhode Island **Method:** Quasi-experimental trial • Experimental group: 3 counties received academic detailing visits • Control group: 2 counties with no intervention **Outcome measures:** Measures of smoking behavior assessed at baseline and at 6, 12, 19, and 24 months **Duration:** 24 months

Description of Educational Method	Findings
* 2 opinion leaders at each site conducted 15-minute academic detailing sessions * On-site pharmacists conducted 2 sessions to discuss physician-specific prescribing patterns in comparison to peer prescribing patterns * A CQI facilitator trained practice leaders in "plan, do, study, act" and the use of real-time data collection	* Academic detailing alone and CQI alone were generally ineffective in improving clinical outcomes * Academic detailing was associated with decreased use of older tricyclics * Use of CQI teams and academic detailing in combination increased percentage of adequately controlled hypertensives
* Resources provided to offices, including patient education resources, pocket cards, and desk prompts * Practice consultants conducted 4-5 visits to offices in the intervention counties	Smokers who resided in intervention areas were more likely to report they had quit smoking than smokers who resided in control areas (OR = 1.35; 95% CI: 0.99-1.83; $P = 0.057$)

continued

TABLE A-2 Continued

Reference	Study Purpose	Sample, Method, Outcome Measures, and Duration
Ilett, K. F., S. Johnson, G. Greenhill, L. Mullen, J. Brockis, C. L. Golledge, and D. B. Reid. 2000. Modification of general practitioner prescribing of antibiotics by use of a therapeutics adviser (academic detailer). *British Journal of Clinical Pharmacology* 49(2):168-173.	Evaluate the use of a clinical pharmacist as an academic detailer to modify antibiotic prescribing by GPs	**Sample:** 112 GPs in Perth, Western Australia **Method:** Randomized controlled trial • Experimental group: academic detailing session • Control group: no intervention **Outcome measures:** Total prescriptions; prescriptions for individual antibiotics before and after the intervention **Duration:** 7 months
Kim, C. S., R. J. Kristopaitis, E. Stone, M. Pelter, M. Sandhu, and S. R. Weingarten. 1999. Physician education and report cards: Do they make the grade? Results from a randomized controlled trial. *American Journal of Medicine* 107(6):556-560.	Determine whether tailored educational interventions can improve the quality of care and lead to better patient satisfaction	**Sample:** 41 primary care physicians who cared for 1,810 patients at a large health maintenance organization **Method:** Randomized controlled trial • Experimental group: ongoing education and academic detailing • Control group: ongoing education **Outcome measures:** Provision of preventive care reported by patients and in medical records; patient satisfaction **Duration:** 2.5 years

Description of Educational Method	Findings
* A panel of experts prepared a best-practice chart of recommended drugs for various infections * A pharmacist visited each prescriber in the experimental group to disseminate the chart and discuss its recommendations	* Academic detailing decreased prescription numbers and costs * Total cost of antibiotics prescribed by doctors in the control group increased by 48% from the pre- to post-intervention periods * Costs for the experimental group increased by only 35%
* All physicians received mailed educational materials that contained overviews of preventive care services * The experimental group received peer-comparison feedback and academic detailing from a pharmacist at 3 separate sessions	* Patient-reported preventive care measures did not align with medical records review data, resulting in an ambiguous effect of education, peer comparison, and academic detailing on preventive services * Education, peer comparison, and academic detailing had modest effects on patient satisfaction

continued

TABLE A-2 Continued

Reference	Study Purpose	Sample, Method, Outcome Measures, and Duration
Mol, P. G. M., J. E. Wieringa, P. V. NannanPanday, R. O. B. Gans, J. E. Degener, M. Laseur, and F. M. Haaijer-Ruskamp. 2005. Improving compliance with hospital antibiotic guidelines: A time-series intervention analysis. *Journal of Antimicrobial Chemotherapy* 55(4): 550-557.	Investigated impact of a 2-phase intervention strategy to improve antimicrobial prescribing compliance with treatment guidelines	**Sample:** 2,869 patients treated with an antimicrobial agent at a teaching hospital in the Netherlands **Method:** Interrupted time-series study **Outcome measures:** Prescribing data collected at baseline, after update of guidelines, and at the conclusion of academic detailing **Duration:** 25 months
Reeve, J. F., G. M. Peterson, R. H. Rumble, and R. Jaffrey. 1999. Programme to improve the use of drugs in older people and involve general practitioners in community education. *Journal of Clinical Pharmacy & Therapeutics* 24(4): 289-297.	Determine the effect of educational materials and academic detailing sessions on GP prescribing patterns for older patients	**Sample:** 13 GPs in Australia **Method:** Cohort study **Outcome measures:** Scores on pre- and post-multiple choice tests; number of prescribed "indicator" medications **Duration:** NA
Siegel, D., J. Lopez, J. Meier, M. K. Goldstein, S. Lee, B. J. Brazill, and M. S. Matalka. 2003. Academic detailing to improve antihypertensive prescribing patterns. *American Journal of Hypertension* 16(6): 508-511.	Determine whether using academic detailing increased practitioner compliance with antihypertensive treatment guidelines	**Sample:** 5 Department of Veterans Affairs (VA) medical facilities **Method:** Quasi-experimental design **Outcome measures:** Antihypertensive prescribing patterns; blood pressures **Duration:** 17 months

Description of Educational Method	Findings
* Sessions with users conducted to improve guidelines * Antimicrobial guidelines were updated and disseminated in paper and electronic formats * Academic detailing was used to improve compliance with the guidelines	* Updating guidelines in collaboration with specialists followed by active dissemination resulted in a significant change in the level of compliance * Academic detailing did not lead to statistically significant changes in already high levels of guideline compliance
* Pharmacist-developed prescribing guidelines discussed at academic detailing sessions * GP-conducted education sessions to interdisciplinary groups of practitioners * Patient-held medication record distributed to elderly patients	* Significant decline in prescribing of psychoactive drugs ($\chi^2 = 4.1$, df = 1, $p < 0.05$) and nonsteroidal anti-inflammatory drugs (NSAIDs) ($\chi^2 = 4.8$, df = 1, $p < 0.05$) * Patient-held medication records were useful in cueing discussions but time-consuming and infrequently used
* 1 pharmacist per VA facility was trained as an academic detailer * Academic detailing included lectures, educational materials, provider profiling (one-on-one meetings), and group meetings	* Prescribing patterns more closely followed national recommendations with use of academic detailing * Changes in prescribing patterns may have resulted from factors other than the intervention

continued

TABLE A-2 Continued

Reference	Study Purpose	Sample, Method, Outcome Measures, and Duration
Simon, S. R., S. R. Majumdar, L. A. Prosser, S. Salem-Schatz, C. Warner, K. Kleinman, I. Miroshnik, and S. B. Soumerai. 2005. Group versus individual academic detailing to improve the use of antihypertensive medications in primary care: A cluster-randomized controlled trial. *American Journal of Medicine* 118(5): 521-528.	Compare group vs. individual academic detailing to increase diuretic and β-blocker use in hypertension	**Sample:** 9,820 patients with newly treated hypertension in a large health maintenance organization **Method:** Cluster randomized controlled trial • Experimental groups: practices received group detailing; individuals received one-on-one academic detailing • Control group: no intervention **Outcome measures:** Rates of diuretic or β-blocker use 1- and 2-years post-intervention; average per-patient cost of antihypertensive medications; rates of hospitalization; per-patient cost of the intervention **Duration:** 3 years
Solomon, D. H., L. Van Houten, R. J. Glynn, L. Baden, K. Curtis, H. Schrager, and J. Avorn. 2001. Academic detailing to improve use of broad-spectrum antibiotics at an academic medical center. *Archives of Internal Medicine* 161(15):1897-1902.	Test the efficacy of academic detailing designed to improve the appropriateness of broad-spectrum antibiotic use	**Sample:** 51 interns and residents in 17 general medicine, oncology, and cardiology services at a teaching hospital **Method:** Randomized controlled trial • Experimental group: academic detailing • Control group: no intervention **Outcome measures:** Number of days that unnecessary levofloxacin or ceftazidime was administered; rate of unnecessary use of levofloxacin or ceftazidime **Duration:** 18 weeks

Description of Educational Method	Findings
* Individual academic detailing entailed a single meeting of a physician-educator with a clinician to address barriers implementing guidelines * Small-group academic detailing with physician "idea champions"	* After 1 year, both individual and group academic detailing improved prescribing compliance by 13% over usual care * By the second year following the interventions, effects had decayed * Group detailing intervention ($3,500) cost less than individual detailing ($5,000); these intervention costs were of similar magnitude to the medication costs savings
* Peer leaders were trained in academic detailing through practice sessions using role play * Academic detailing targeted to interns and residents who wrote an unnecessary order	* Length of stay, intensive care unit transfers, readmission rates, and in-hospital death rates were similar in both groups * 37% reduction in days of unnecessary antibiotic use ($p < 0.001$) * Rate of unnecessary use of the 2 target antibiotics reduced by 41% (95% CI: 44-78%, $p < 0.001$)

continued

TABLE A-2 Continued

Reference	Study Purpose	Sample, Method, Outcome Measures, and Duration
Van Eijk, M. E. C., J. Avorn, A. J. Porsius, and A. De Boer. 2001. Reducing prescribing of highly anticholinergic antidepressants for elderly people: Randomised trial of group versus individual academic detailing. *British Medical Journal* 322(7287):654-657.	Compare effect of individual vs. group academic detailing on prescribing of highly anticholinergic antidepressants in elderly people	**Sample:** 190 GPs and 37 pharmacists in 21 peer-review groups in the Netherlands **Method:** Randomized controlled trial • Experimental groups: individual academic detailing; group academic detailing • Control group: no intervention **Outcome measure:** Incidence rates calculated as the number of elderly people with new prescriptions of highly anticholinergic antidepressants **Duration:** NA
Wong, R. Y., and P. E. Lee. 2004. Teaching physicians geriatric principles: A randomized control trial on academic detailing plus printed materials versus printed materials only. *Journals of Gerontology Series A-Biological Sciences & Medical Sciences* 59(10):1036-1040.	Compare the effectiveness of academic detailing with printed materials on promoting geriatric knowledge among physicians	**Sample:** 19 post-graduate trainees (residents and fellows) in British Columbia, Canada **Method:** Randomized controlled trial • Experimental group: printed materials and academic detailing • Control group: printed materials **Outcome measures:** Scores on pre and post multiple choice tests **Duration:** 12 months

Description of Educational Method	Findings
* A peer educator met individually with GPs to discuss guidelines and prescribing patterns from the past year * Group academic detailing sessions were similar to the individual sessions and included group and individual performance data	* Individual and group academic detailing improved the clinical appropriateness of prescribing behavior * Patients in both groups more likely to receive drugs that were less anticholinergic
15-minute face-to-face educational outreach with a specialist in geriatric medicine	Academic detailing plus printed educational materials demonstrated a trend toward increased knowledge retention (1.1 ± 1.3) compared with printed materials alone (0.0 ± 1.1, $p = 0.053$)

continued

TABLE A-2 Continued

Reference	Study Purpose	Sample, Method, Outcome Measures, and Duration
Simulation		
Crofts, J. F., C. Bartlett, D. Ellis, L. P. Hunt, R. Fox, and T. J. Draycott. 2006. Training for shoulder dystocia: A trial of simulation using low-fidelity and high-fidelity mannequins. *Obstetrics and Gynecology* 108(6):1477-1485.	* Evaluate the effectiveness of simulation training for shoulder dystocia management * Compare training using a high-fidelity mannequin with training using a traditional mannequin	**Sample:** 45 physicians and 95 midwives **Method:** Randomized controlled trial • Experimental group: training with high-fidelity mannequins • Control group: training with traditional, low-fidelity mannequins **Outcome measures:** Pre- and post-training delivery, head-to-body delivery time, use of appropriate actions, force applied, and communication **Duration:** NA
Gerson, L. B., and J. Van Dam. 2003. A prospective randomized trial comparing a virtual reality simulator to bedside teaching for training in sigmoidoscopy. *Endoscopy* 35(7):569-575.	Compare the exclusive use of a virtual reality endoscopy simulator with bedside teaching for training in sigmoidoscopy	**Sample:** 16 internal medicine residents at an academic medical center **Method:** Prospective randomized controlled trial • Experimental group: training using a virtual reality simulator • Control group: bedside teaching **Outcome measures:** Score on 5 endoscopic evaluations based on procedure duration, completion, ability to perform retroflexion, and level of patient comfort or discomfort **Duration:** 10 months

Description of Educational Method	Findings
* High-fidelity mannequin training incorporated force perception and occurred at a simulation center * Low-fidelity mannequin training occurred at local hospitals	* Both high- and low-fidelity simulation were associated with improved successful deliveries pre- and post-training (42.9% vs. 83.3%, p < 0.001) * Training with high-fidelity mannequins was associated with a higher successful delivery rate than the control (94% vs. 72%; OR: 6.53; 95% CI: 2.05-20.81; p = 0.02)
Residents had unlimited use of a virtual reality simulator that included • Didactic modules and practice cases • Virtual patients that complained when appropriate • Critique provided by simulator • No bedside teaching	* Simulator group had more difficulty with initial endoscope insertion and endoscope negotiation than control group residents * Simulator group less likely to be able to perform retroflexion (mean score = 2.9) than the control group residents (mean score = 3.8) (p < 0.001)

continued

TABLE A-2 Continued

Reference	Study Purpose	Sample, Method, Outcome Measures, and Duration
Gordon, D. L., S. B. Issenberg, M. S. Gordon, D. Lacombe, W. C. McGaghie, and E. R. Petrusa. 2005. Stroke training of prehospital providers: An example of simulation-enhanced blended learning and evaluation. *Medical Teacher* 27(2):114-121.	Assess the effectiveness of a stroke course that incorporates didactic lectures, tabletop exercises, small-group sessions, and standardized patients (a type of simulation used to develop communication, interpersonal, and psychomotor skills)	**Sample:** 73 pre-hospital paraprofessionals participating in a stroke class **Method:** Cohort study with a pre- and post-intervention design **Outcome measures:** Scores on a pre- and post-multiple choice test; scores on 4 case scenarios as determined by clinician raters **Duration:** 9 months
Grantcharov, T. P., V. B. Kristiansen, J. Bendix, L. Bardram, J. Rosenberg, and P. Funch-Jensen. 2004. Randomized clinical trial of virtual reality simulation for laparoscopic skills training. *British Journal of Surgery* 91(2):146-150.	Examine the impact of virtual reality simulation on improvement of psychomotor skills relevant to the performance of laparoscopic cholecystectomy	**Sample:** 16 surgical trainees **Method:** Randomized controlled trial • Experimental group: virtual reality training • Control group: no training **Outcome measures:** Baseline and post-intervention time to complete the procedure, error score, and economy-of-movement score **Duration:** 2 years
Quinn, F., P. Keogh, A. McDonald, and D. Hussey. 2003. A study comparing the effectiveness of conventional training and virtual reality simulation in the skills acquisition of junior dental students. *European Journal of Dental Education: Official Journal of the Association for Dental Education in Europe* 7(4):164-169.	Measure the effectiveness of exclusive use of a virtual reality simulator in the training of operative dentistry	**Sample:** 20 second-year dental undergraduate students in Dublin, Ireland **Method:** Randomized controlled trial • Experimental group: trained solely by virtual reality • Control group: conventional training using a combination of virtual reality and clinical instruction **Outcome measures:** Assessment on 2 class-1 cavities **Duration:** NA

Description of Educational Method	Findings
Participants evaluated 2 standardized patients before the stroke course and 2 different standardized patients after the stroke course	Mean scores on case scenarios improved significantly (85.4%) from the pre-test (53.9%) ($p < 0.0001$)
Experimental group participated in 10 repetitions of each of 6 tasks on a virtual reality surgical simulator	* Experimental group performed laparoscopic surgery significantly faster than control group ($p = 0.021$) * Experimental group showed significantly greater improvement in economy-of-movement scores ($p = 0.003$)
* Both groups carried out procedures on virtual reality-based training units * The control group received feedback and evaluation from a clinical instructor * The experimental group received real-time feedback and software evaluation from the virtual reality simulator	* Group trained exclusively on the virtual reality simulator scored worse on cavity assessment * 84% of participants did not believe exclusive virtual reality training could replace conventional training

continued

TABLE A-2 Continued

Reference	Study Purpose	Sample, Method, Outcome Measures, and Duration
Schwid, H. A., G. A. Rooke, P. Michalowski, and B. K. Ross. 2001. Screen-based anesthesia simulation with debriefing improves performance in a mannequin-based anesthesia simulator. *Teaching & Learning in Medicine* 13(2):92-96.	Measure the effectiveness of screen-based simulator training with debriefing on the response to simulated anesthetic critical incidents	**Sample:** 21 first-year clinical anesthesia residents **Method:** Randomized controlled trial • Experimental group: screen-based simulator • Control group: traditional handout **Outcome measures:** Quantitative scoring on residents' management of 4 standardized scenarios in a mannequin-based simulator **Duration:** 2 years
Triola, M., H. Feldman, A. L. Kalet, S. Zabar, E. K. Kachur, C. Gillespie, M. Anderson, C. Griesser, and M. Lipkin. 2006. A randomized trial of teaching clinical skills using virtual and live standardized patients. *Journal of General Internal Medicine* 21(5):424-429.	Assess the educational effectiveness of computer-based virtual patients compared to standardized patients	**Sample:** 55 health care providers (RNs and physicians) **Method:** Randomized controlled trial • Experimental group: training using 2 live, standardized patients and 2 virtual (web-based) cases • Control group: training using 4 live, standardized patients **Outcome measures:** Knowledge and diagnostic scores assessed through clinical vignettes **Duration:** 1 day

Description of Educational Method	Findings
* The simulator used a graphical interface and an automated record system to produce a detailed record of the simulated case * The program included learning objectives and diagnostic and treatment suggestions	Residents who managed anesthetic problems using a screen-based simulator handled emergencies in a mannequin-based simulator (52.6 ± 9.9) better than residents who studied a handout (43.4 ± 5.9, $p = 0.004$)
* Virtual (web-based) standardized cases were conducted individually at a computer * Live, standardized patient cases were faculty-facilitated, small-group sessions	* Experimental and control groups scored the same in preparedness to respond ($p = 0.61$), to screen ($p = 0.79$), and to care ($p = 0.055$) for patients * Improvement in diagnostic abilities were equivalent in both groups ($p = 0.054$)

continued

TABLE A-2 Continued

Reference	Study Purpose	Sample, Method, Outcome Measures, and Duration
Reminders		
Cannon, D. S., and S. N. Allen. 2000. A comparison of the effects of computer and manual reminders on compliance with a mental health clinical practice guideline. *Journal of the American Medical Informatics Association* 7(2):196-203.	Evaluate the relative effectiveness of computer and manual reminder systems on the implementation of clinical practice guidelines	**Sample:** 78 outpatients and 4 senior clinicians at an urban VA Medical Center **Method:** Randomized controlled trial • Experimental group: computer reminder system • Control group: paper checklists **Outcome measures:** Screening rates for mood disorder; completeness of the documentation of diagnostic criteria for patients with a major depressive disorder **Duration:** 9 months
Chen, P., M. J. Tanasijevic, R. A. Schoenenberger, J. Fiskio, G. J. Kuperman, and D. W. Bates. 2003. A computer-based intervention for improving the appropriateness of antiepileptic drug level monitoring. *American Journal of Clinical Pathology* 119(3):432-438.	* Evaluate an automated, activity-based reminder designed to reduce inappropriate ordering behavior * Determine the long-term benefit of continuous implementation of the reminder system	**Sample:** 1,646 serum antiepileptic drug (AED) test orders placed at a teaching hospital **Method:** 2-phase randomized controlled trial • Phase 1: Experimental group: reminders Control group: no intervention • Phase 2: After 3 months, all physicians received reminders **Outcome measures:** Total number of AED orders; proportion of inappropriate orders; proportion of redundant orders **Duration:** 4 years

Description of Educational Method	Findings
* The CaseWalker computer reminder system generated reminders to screen patients for mood disorders * The CaseWalker system presented and scored diagnostic criteria for major depressive disorders and created progress notes	* Computerized reminders, compared with the paper checklist, resulted in a higher screening rate for mood disorder (86.5% vs. 61%, $p = 0.008$) * Computerized reminders resulted in a higher rate of complete documentation of diagnostic criteria (100% vs. 5.6%, $p < 0.001$)
Educational messages reminded physicians of clinical guidelines when test orders may have been inappropriate or redundant	* During a 3-month period after implementation, 13% of ordered tests were canceled following computerized reminders; for orders appearing redundant, 27% cancellation rate * Cancellation rate sustained after 4 years * 19.5% decrease in AED testing volume despite a 19.3% increase in overall chemistry test volume

continued

TABLE A-2 Continued

Reference	Study Purpose	Sample, Method, Outcome Measures, and Duration
Demakis, J. G., C. Beauchamp, W. L. Cull, R. Denwood, S. A. Eisen, R. Lofgren, K. Nichol, J. Woolliscroft, and W. G. Henderson. 2000. Improving residents' compliance with standards of ambulatory care: Results from the VA cooperative study on computerized reminders. *Journal of the American Medical Association* 284(11):1411-1416.	Examine whether a computerized reminder system operating in multiple VA ambulatory care clinics improves resident physician compliance with standards of ambulatory care	**Sample:** 275 resident physicians caring for 12,989 patients at 12 VA medical centers **Method:** Clinical trial • Experimental group: reminders • Control group: no intervention **Outcome measures:** Compliance with 13 standards of care, tracked using hospital databases and encounter forms **Duration:** 17 months
Dexter, P. R., S. Perkins, J. Marc Overhage, K. Maharry, R. B. Kohler, and C. J. McDonald. 2001. A computerized reminder system to increase the use of preventive care for hospitalized patients. *New England Journal of Medicine* 345(13):965-970.	Determine the effects of computerized reminders on the rates at which 4 preventive therapies were ordered for inpatients	**Sample:** 8 independent staff teams on the general medicine ward and 6,371 patients at an urban hospital **Method:** Randomized controlled trial • Experimental group: reminders • Control group: no intervention **Outcome measures:** Ordering rates for pneumococcal vaccination, influenza vaccination, prophylactic heparin, and prophylactic aspirin **Duration:** 18 months

Description of Educational Method	Findings
* All residents attended a 1-hour session to discuss standards of care * Residents in the experimental group had a training session to introduce them to the reminder system	* Experimental group had statistically significant higher rates of compliance than the control group for all care standards combined (58.8% vs. 53.5%; OR = 1.24; 95% CI) * Percentage of compliance in the experimental group declined over the course of the study, even though the reminders remained active
* Computer-based order-entry work stations provided clinical decision support through rule-based reminders * Physicians could accept or reject the reminders	Computerized reminders resulted in higher adjusted ordering rates for • Pneumococcal vaccination (35.8% vs. 0.8%, $p < 0.001$) • Influenza vaccination (51.4% vs. 1.0%, $p < 0.001$) • Prophylactic heparin (32.3% vs. 18.9%, $p < 0.001$) • Prophylactic aspirin (36.4% vs. 27.6%, $p < 0.001$)

continued

TABLE A-2 Continued

Reference	Study Purpose	Sample, Method, Outcome Measures, and Duration
Dexter, P. R., F. D. Wolinsky, G. P. Gramelspacher, X. H. Zhou, G. J. Eckert, M. Waisburd, and W. M. Tierney. 1998. Effectiveness of computer-generated reminders for increasing discussions about advance directives and completion of advance directive forms: A randomized, controlled trial. *Annals of Internal Medicine* 128(2): 102-110.	* Determine the effects of computer-generated reminders to physicians on the frequency of advanced directive discussions between patients and their primary caregivers * Determine the effects of computer-generated reminders to physicians on consequent establishment of advanced directives	**Sample:** 1,009 patients and 147 primary care physicians at an outpatient general medicine practice **Method:** Randomized controlled trial • Experimental group: computerized reminders • Control group: no intervention **Outcome measures:** Discussion about advanced directives determined by patient interview; completed advanced directive forms **Duration:** 9 months
Gill, J. M., and A. M. Saldarriaga. 2000. The impact of a computerized physician reminder and a mailed patient reminder on influenza immunizations for older patients. *Delaware Medical Journal* 72(10):425-430.	Examine the impact of a computer physician reminder in combination with a mailed patient reminder on the rate of influenza vaccinations for older adults	**Sample:** 344 patients 65 years and older in a large family medicine office **Method:** Retrospective cohort study **Outcome measures:** Rates of receipt of influenza immunization compared to the year before and after the interventions were implemented **Duration:** 2 years

Description of Educational Method	Findings
* Advanced directive forms placed in the offices of all participating physicians * Physician-investigators presented the concepts of advanced directives at grand rounds and face-to-face meetings with all physicians * Experimental group physicians received reminders regarding advanced directive discussions	* Physicians who received reminders discussed advanced directives with more patients (24%) than control group physicians (4%) (OR = 7.7, 95% CI: 3.4-18, $p < 0.001$) * Experimental group completed advanced directives with 15% of patients compared to 4% completion in control group (OR = 7.0, 95% CI: 2.9-17, $p < 0.001$)
* An electronic patient record system generated automatic reminders to the physician if the immunization had not been completed * A mailed patient reminder was sent to encourage patients to schedule appointments for the immunization	Influenza immunization rates increase from 50.4% before the interventions to 61.6% after the intervention ($p < 0.001$)

continued

TABLE A-2 Continued

Reference	Study Purpose	Sample, Method, Outcome Measures, and Duration
Hung, C. S., J. W. Lin, J. J. Hwang, R. Y. Tsai, and A. T. Li. 2008. Using paper chart based clinical reminders to improve guideline adherence to lipid management. *Journal of Evaluation in Clinical Practice* 14(5):861-866.	Apply a paper-based clinical reminder to improve the adherence to lipid guidelines	**Sample:** 198 patients with coronary heart diseases at a university hospital in Taiwan **Method:** Randomized controlled trial • Experimental group: clinical reminder stamped on the paper chart • Control group: no intervention **Outcome measures:** New lipid-lowering therapy subscription; composite result of lipid-lowering therapy or lipid profile checkup **Duration:** 6 months
Iliadis, E. A., L. W. Klein, B. J. Vandenberg, D. Spokas, T. Hursey, J. E. Parrillo, and J. E. Calvin. 1999. Clinical practice guidelines in unstable angina improve clinical outcomes by assuring early intensive medical treatment. *Journal of the American College of Cardiology* 34(6): 1689-1695.	* Determine the influence of clinical practice guidelines on treatment patterns and clinical outcomes in unstable angina * Determine the effectiveness of guideline reminders on implementing practice guidelines	**Sample:** 519 patients with unstable angina at an academic medical center **Method:** Interrupted time-series design • Experimental group: admitted after institution of guideline reminders • Control group: admitted before publication of guidelines **Outcome measures:** Pharmaceutical treatments rendered; diagnostic or therapeutic procedures performed; major cardiac complications **Duration:** 3.5 years

Description of Educational Method	Findings
* In the experimental group, a reminder was stamped in each medical chart * The reminder indicated the current policy of statin reimbursement	* No difference at the end of 6 months regarding lipid-lowering therapy subscription (OR = 1.70, p = 0.248, 95% CI: 0.69-4.19) * Composite result of lipid-lowering therapy or lipid profile checkup significantly higher in the experimental group (OR = 2.81, p = 0.001, 95% CI: 1.57-5.04)
Dissemination of guidelines was ensured by a grand rounds lecture and by posting guideline reminders on all of the experimental group's charts	* Experimental group patients received β-blockers (p = 0.008), aspirin, and coronary angiography (p = 0.001) earlier than control group patients * Experimental group patients experienced recurrent angina (29% vs. 54%) and myocardial infarction or death less frequently (3% vs. 9%, p = 0.028) than control group patients

continued

TABLE A-2 Continued

Reference	Study Purpose	Sample, Method, Outcome Measures, and Duration
Kitahata, M. M., P. W. Dillingham, N. Chaiyakunapruk, S. E. Buskin, J. L. Jones, R. D. Harrington, T. M. Hooton, and K. K. Holmes. 2003. Electronic human immunodeficiency virus (HIV) clinical reminder system improves adherence to practice guidelines among the University of Washington HIV study cohort. *Clinical Infectious Diseases* 36(6):803-811.	Examine adherence to HIV practice guidelines before and after implementation of an electronic clinical reminder system	**Sample:** 1,204 HIV-infected patients and 41 clinicians (physicians, nurse practitioners, and physician assistants) at an HIV clinic in an academic medical center **Method:** Prospective before-and-after study **Outcome measures:** Proportion of patients in care who undergo (1) monitoring of CD4 cell count, (2) HIV-1 RNA level, (3) prophylaxis for pneumocystis pneumonia, (4) MAC prophylaxis, (5) tuberculin skin testing, (6) cervical Pap smears, and (7) serological screening **Duration:** 5 years
Koide, D., K. Ohe, D. Ross-Degnan, and S. Kaihara. 2000. Computerized reminders to monitor liver function to improve the use of etretinate. *International Journal of Medical Informatics* 57(1):11-19.	Determine whether computerized reminders during the process of prescribing can improve the use of drugs requiring prior laboratory testing	**Sample:** 1,024 prescriptions prescribed for 111 patients at a teaching hospital in Tokyo, Japan **Method:** Interrupted time-series design to compare a pre-intervention period and a post-intervention period **Outcome measures:** Change in proportion of appropriate prescribing; frequency of severe hepatotoxicity between pre- and post-intervention **Duration:** 2 years

Description of Educational Method	Findings
An HIV disease-specific electronic medical record (EMR) enhancement provided clinicians with access to patient-specific information and a clinical reminder system	* More than 90% of patients received CD4 cell count and HIV-1 RNA level monitoring both before and after the intervention * Patients were significantly more likely to receive prophylaxis (hazard ratio = 3.84; 95% CI, 1.58-9.31; $p = 0.03$), to undergo cervical cancer screening (OR = 2.09; 95% CI, 1.04-4.16; $p = 0.04$), and to undergo serological screening (OR = 1.86; 95% CI, 1.05-3.27; $p = 0.03$) after the reminders were implemented
* Computer alerts when physicians submit inappropriate prescriptions * The physician can choose to proceed despite the alert or to cancel the prescription	* Appropriate prescriptions increased from 25.9% (127/491) in the pre-intervention period to 66.2% (353/533) in the post-intervention period ($p < 0.0001$)

continued

TABLE A-2 Continued

Reference	Study Purpose	Sample, Method, Outcome Measures, and Duration
Morgan, M. M., J. Goodson, and G. O. Barnett. 1998. Long-term changes in compliance with clinical guidelines through computer-based reminders. *Proceedings of the American Medical Informatics Association Annual Fall Symposium* 493-497.	* Evaluate the effectiveness of computer-based reminders in improving compliance with preventive medicine screening guidelines * Examine the long-term impact of these reminders	**Sample:** 24,200 patients and 20 primary care physicians **Method:** Ecologic study with a 12-month period prior to introduction of reminders, a 12-month period after the reminders were in place, and 5 years later **Outcome measures:** Changes in compliance rates for preventive screenings **Duration:** 6 years
Nilasena, D. S., and M. J. Lincoln. 1995. A computer-generated reminder system improves physician compliance with diabetes preventive care guidelines. *Proceedings of the Annual Symposium on Computer Applications in Medical Care* 640-645.	Evaluate the use of computerized reminders for preventive care in diabetes	**Sample:** 35 internal medicine residents **Method:** Randomized controlled trial • Experimental group: detailed patient-specific reports and encounter forms • Control group: blank encounter forms **Outcome measure:** Average compliance score of all patients seen by a resident (compliance score based on the number of items completed in accordance with the guidelines divided by the total number of items recommended for the patient) **Duration:** 6 months

Description of Educational Method	Findings
* Physicians were given a health maintenance report of preventive screening items at each patient visit * EMR system was programmed to integrate 13 clinical guidelines	* Mean performance on 10 out of 13 health maintenance measures improved in the year following the integrated guideline report * 5 years after introduction, improvement in mean performance persisted on 7 out of 13 measures and compliance improved for 1 additional measure
* Diabetes guidelines and encounter forms were incorporated in a computer program that served as a longitudinal patient database for storing clinical information * The computer program outputs a health maintenance report for the physician, and the report is placed on the patient's chart * Clinical alerts about high-risk aspects of the patient's profile are presented	Compliance with recommended care significantly improved in both the experimental group (38% at baseline, 54.9% at follow-up) and the control group (34.6% at baseline, 51% at follow-up)

continued

TABLE A-2 Continued

Reference	Study Purpose	Sample, Method, Outcome Measures, and Duration
Rhew, D. C., P. A. Glassman, and M. B. Goetz. 1999. Improving pneumococcal vaccine rates. Nurse protocols versus clinical reminders. *Journal of General Internal Medicine* 14(6):351-356.	Compare the effectiveness of 3 interventions designed to improve the pneumococcal vaccination rate by nurses	**Sample:** 3,502 outpatients and 3 nursing teams at a VA ambulatory care clinic **Method:** Prospective controlled trial • Experimental groups: comparative feedback and clinician reminders (Team A); compliance reminders and clinician reminders (Team B) • Control group: clinical reminders **Outcome measure:** Vaccination rates **Duration:** 12 weeks
Sarasin, F. P., M. L. Maschiangelo, M. D. Schaller, C. Heliot, S. Mischler, and J. M. Gaspoz. 1999. Successful implementation of guidelines for encouraging the use of beta blockers in patients after acute myocardial infarction. *American Journal of Medicine* 106(5):499-505.	Assess whether implementation of guidelines increases the prescription of β-blockers recommended for secondary prevention after acute myocardial infarction	**Sample:** 355 patients discharged after recovery from myocardial infarction from a teaching hospital in Geneva, Switzerland **Method:** Ecologic study with 12-month control period and a 6-month guideline implementation period; a neighboring public teaching hospital was used as a comparison **Outcome measures:** Prescription patterns for nitrates, β-blockers, combined β-blockers and angiotensin-converting enzyme (ACE) inhibitors, and ACE inhibitors alone; physician attitude survey **Duration:** 18 months

Description of Educational Method	Findings
* Team A nurses received comparative feedback information on their vaccine rates relative to those of Team B nurses * Team B nurses received reminders to vaccinate but no information on vaccination rates * Nurses in all groups received clinician reminders	Vaccination rates for comparative feedback group and compliance reminder group were significantly higher than the 5% vaccination rate for the control group ($p < 0.001$)
* Short advisory statements regarding drug therapies were presented and distributed to all internal medicine and cardiology physicians * Adherence was encouraged during large group meetings * Guidelines were placed in the charts of all patients diagnosed with acute myocardial infarction	Implementation of guidelines significantly associated with prescription of β-blockers at discharge (OR = 10; 95% CI: 3.2-33; $p < 0.001$)

continued

TABLE A-2 Continued

Reference	Study Purpose	Sample, Method, Outcome Measures, and Duration
Tang, P. C., M. P. Larosa, C. Newcomb, and S. M. Gorden. 1999. Measuring the effects of reminders for outpatient influenza immunizations at the point of clinical opportunity. *Journal of the American Medical Informatics Association* 6(2):115-121.	Evaluate the influence of computer-based reminders about influenza vaccination on the behavior of individual clinicians at each clinical opportunity	**Sample:** 23 physicians and 629 patients at an internal medicine clinic at an academic medical center **Method:** Cohort study • Experimental group: computer-based patient record system that generated reminders • Control group: traditional paper records **Outcome measures:** Compliance with a guideline for influenza vaccination behavior for eligible patients as evidenced by ordering of the vaccine, patient counseling, or verification that the patient had received the vaccine elsewhere **Duration:** 4 years
Walker, N. M., K. L. Mandell, and J. Tsevat. 1999. Use of chart reminders for physicians to promote discussion of advance directives in patients with AIDS. *AIDS Care* 11(3):345-353.	Determine if use of a physician chart reminder improves the rate of physician-initiated discussion and subsequent completion of advanced directives in patients with AIDS	**Sample:** 74 patients with AIDS and 10 primary care physicians at a university-based hospital clinic **Method:** Controlled trial • Experimental group: chart reminders • Control group: no intervention **Outcome measures:** Rate of documentation of discussion of advanced directives and rate of completion of an advanced directive **Duration:** 6 months

Description of Educational Method	Findings
Rule-based clinical reminders appeared on the electronic chart of a patient eligible for a recommended intervention	Compliance rates for computer-based record users increased 78% from baseline ($p < 0.001$) whereas rates for paper record users did not change significantly ($p = 0.18$)
Chart reminders were placed on medical records of experimental group patients at each clinic visit	* 12 out of 39 (31%) experimental group patients and 3 out of 35 (9%, $p = 0.02$) control group patients discussed advanced directives with physicians * More subjects in experimental group completed advanced directives (28% vs. 9%, $p = 0.03$)

continued

TABLE A-2 Continued

Reference	Study Purpose	Sample, Method, Outcome Measures, and Duration
Weingarten, S. R., M. S. Riedinger, L. Conner, T. H. Lee, I. Hoffman, B. Johnson, and A. G. Ellrodt. 1994. Practice guidelines and reminders to reduce duration of hospital stay for patients with chest pain: An interventional trial. *Annals of Internal Medicine* 120(4):257-263.	Evaluate the acceptability, safety, and efficacy of practice guidelines for patients admitted to coronary care and intermediate care units	**Sample:** 375 patients with chest pain and 155 primary physicians at an academic medical center **Method:** Prospective, controlled clinical trial • Experimental group: guideline reminders • Control group: no intervention **Outcome measures:** Patient instability at discharge; patient survival, hospital readmission, and other problems 1-month post-discharge; patient health perceptions; patient rating of the quality of information received at discharge; total costs (direct and indirect) **Duration:** 12 months

Protocols and Guidelines

| Dexter, P. R., S. M. Perkins, K. S. Maharry, K. Jones, and C. J. McDonald. 2004. Inpatient computer-based standing orders vs. physician reminders to increase influenza and pneumococcal vaccination rates: A randomized trial. *Journal of the American Medical Association* 292(19):2366-2371. | Determine the effects of computerized physician standing orders compared with physician reminders on inpatient vaccination rates | **Sample:** 3,777 general medicine patients discharged during a 14-month period from an urban teaching hospital **Method:** Randomized controlled trial
• Experimental group: reminder team
• Control group: standing-order team
Outcome measures: Vaccine administration **Duration:** 14 months |

Description of Educational Method	Findings
Physicians received concurrent, personalized written and verbal reminders regarding a guideline that recommended a 2-day hospital stay for patients with chest pain who were at low risk for complications	* Use of practice guidelines with concurrent reminders was associated with a 50-69% increase in guideline compliance ($p < 0.001$) and a decrease in length of stay from 3.54 ± 4.1 to 2.63 ± 3.0 days (95% CI) * Intervention associated with a total cost reduction of $1,397 per patient (CI: $176-$2,618; $p = 0.03$) * No significant difference found in complication rates, patient health status, or patient satisfaction
* For eligible patients in the standing order group, a computer system automatically produced a vaccine order at the time of discharge; nurses were authorized to administer vaccines in response to standing orders * For eligible patients in the reminder group, a computer system produced a pop-up message with orders each time a physician began a daily order entry session	* Patients with standing orders received an influenza vaccine significantly more often (42%) than those with reminders (30%) ($p < 0.001$) * Patients with standing orders received a pneumococcal vaccine significantly more often (51%) than those with reminders (31%) ($p < 0.001$)

continued

TABLE A-2 Continued

Reference	Study Purpose	Sample, Method, Outcome Measures, and Duration
Fakhry, S. M., A. L. Trask, M. A. Waller, and D. D. Watts. 2004. Management of brain-injured patients by an evidence-based medicine protocol improves outcomes and decreases hospital charges. *Journal of Trauma* 56(3):492-499.	Determine whether management of traumatic brain injury (TBI) patients according to established guidelines would reduce mortality, length of stay, charges, and disability	**Sample:** 830 patients with TBI **Method:** Time trend analysis • Experimental groups: period of low guideline compliance; period of high guideline compliance • Control group: pre-guideline period **Outcome measures:** Mortality; intensive care unit days; total hospital days; total charges; Rancho Los Amigos Scores; Glasgow Outcome Scale scores **Duration:** 9 years

Audit and Feedback

Lobach, D. F. 1996. Electronically distributed, computer-generated, individualized feedback enhances the use of a computerized practice guideline. *Proceedings of the American Medical Informatics Association Annual Fall Symposium* 493-497.	Test the hypothesis that computer-generated, individualized feedback regarding adherence to care guidelines will significantly improve clinician compliance with guideline recommendations	**Sample:** 45 primary care clinicians at a clinic affiliated with an academic medical center **Method:** Randomized controlled trial • Experimental group: biweekly e-mail with feedback on guideline compliance • Control group: no intervention **Outcome measures:** Compliance with guideline recommendations for diabetic patients **Duration:** 12 weeks

Description of Educational Method	Findings
* Standard orders were developed based on established guidelines * Guidelines were implemented by trauma service team leaders	* From the pre-guideline period to the period of high compliance, ICU stay was reduced by 1.8 days ($p = 0.021$) and hospital stay by 5.4 days ($p < 0.001$) * Overall mortality rate was reduced from pre-guideline period (17.8%) to period of high compliance (13.8%), but the result was not statistically significant ($p > 0.05$) * On Glasgow Outcome Scale score, 61.5% of patients in high compliance period had a "good recovery" or "moderate disability" compared with 43.3% in pre-guideline period ($p < 0.001$)
* The study site used a computer-based patient record that runs a computer-assisted management protocol, which incorporates guidelines for diabetes mellitus on paper encounter forms * E-mail was used to transmit clinical information	Experimental group had significantly higher guideline compliance (35%) than control group (6.1%) ($p < 0.01$)

continued

TABLE A-2 Continued

Reference	Study Purpose	Sample, Method, Outcome Measures, and Duration
Multifaceted Interventions		
Baker, R., A. Farooqi, C. Tait, and S. Walsh. 1997. Randomised controlled trial of reminders to enhance the impact of audit in general practice on management of patients who use benzodiazepines. *Quality in Health Care* 6(1):14-18.	Determine whether reminder cards in medical records enhance the effectiveness of audit and feedback in improving the care of patients with long-term benzodiazepine drugs	**Sample:** 742 patients taking a benzodiazepine in 18 general practices in Leicestershire, UK **Method:** Randomized controlled trial • Experimental group: feedback plus reminder cards • Control group: feedback **Outcome measures:** Number of patients whose care complies with each of 5 criteria **Duration:** NA
Cleland, J. A., J. M. Fritz, G. P. Brennan, and J. Magel. 2009. Does continuing education improve physical therapists' effectiveness in treating neck pain? A randomized clinical trial. *Physical Therapy* 89(1):38-47.	Investigate the effectiveness of an ongoing educational intervention for improving the outcomes for patients with neck pain	**Sample:** 19 physical therapists from 11 clinical sites in an integrated health system **Method:** Randomized controlled trial • Experimental group: ongoing CE • Control group: no further education **Outcome measures:** All patients treated by the physical therapists completed the Neck Disability Index and a pain rating scale before and after the ongoing intervention **Duration:** 7 weeks

Description of Educational Method	Findings
* All practices received a copy of audit criteria justifying "must do" and "should do" priorities * All practices received feedback comparing their performance to the criteria and to other practices * The group receiving reminders had the reminders placed in the records of long-term benzodiazepine users	* Number of patients whose care complied with criteria rose after the interventions (OR: 1.46, 95% CI: 1.32-5.21) * The increase was not statistically greater in practices receiving feedback plus reminders than in those receiving only feedback
* 2-day course on management of neck pain (for both control and experimental groups) * 2 1.5-hour meetings to review the 2-day course, discuss management of specific cases, and co-treat a patient with neck pain in the therapist's own setting (experimental group only)	* Patients treated by experimental group therapists experienced significantly greater reduction in disability during study period than those treated by therapists who did not receive ongoing training (mean difference = 4.2 points) * Pain ratings did not differ for patients treated by the 2 groups

continued

TABLE A-2 Continued

Reference	Study Purpose	Sample, Method, Outcome Measures, and Duration
Fjortoft, N. F., and A. H. Schwartz. 2003. Evaluation of a pharmacy continuing education program: Long-term learning outcomes and changes in practice behaviors. *American Journal of Pharmaceutical Education* 67(2).	Assess the long-term outcomes from a 3-month, curriculum-based pharmacy CE program on lipid management and hypertension services	**Sample:** 46 participants in a pharmacy continuing education course **Method:** Cohort study with a pre- and post-test design **Outcome measure:** Survey responses assessing participant knowledge on cognitive and psychomotor concepts; time spent providing clinical services **Duration:** 3 months
Gonzales, R., J. F. Steiner, A. Lum, and P. H. Barrett, Jr. 1999. Decreasing antibiotic use in ambulatory practice: Impact of a multidimensional intervention on the treatment of uncomplicated acute bronchitis in adults. *Journal of the American Medical Association* 281(16):1512-1519.	Decrease total antibiotic use for uncomplicated acute bronchitis in adults	**Sample:** 93 clinicians (physicians, physician assistants, nurse practitioners, RNs) and 4,489 patients in 6 primary care practices **Method:** Prospective, nonrandomized controlled trial with baseline and study periods • Experimental groups: full intervention; partial intervention • Control group: no intervention **Outcome measures:** Antibiotic prescriptions for uncomplicated acute bronchitis during baseline and study periods **Duration:** 15 months
Hobma, S. O., P. M. Ram, F. van Merode, C. P. M. van der Vleuten, and R. P. T. M. Grol. 2004. Feasibility, appreciation and costs of a tailored continuing professional development approach for general practitioners. *Quality in Primary Care* 12(4):271-278.	Study the feasibility and appreciation of a tailored continuing professional development (CPD) method in which GPs work in small groups to improve demonstrated deficiencies	**Sample:** 43 GPs in the Netherlands **Method:** Cohort study **Outcome measures:** Participation rates; costs per participant based on time invested by support staff, costs of materials, and time dedicated to the intervention; participant appreciation by self-reported Likert scale **Duration:** 11 months

Description of Educational Method	Findings
* Self-study materials * 3 live, interactive workshops with case discussion and physical assessment	* Improvements in participant knowledge base and skill were observed between pre- and post-survey administration * No change in percentage of time spent providing clinical services observed at 6 months or at 12 months
* 2 practices received house- and office-based patient education materials, clinician education, practice-profiling, and academic detailing (full intervention) * 2 practices received only office-based patient education materials (partial intervention)	* Substantial decline in antibiotic prescription rates at the full intervention site (from 74% to 48%, $p = 0.003$) but no statistically significant change at the control and partial intervention sites * Compared with control sites, nonantibiotic prescriptions (cough suppressants, analgesics) and return office visits were not significantly different for intervention sites
*Assessment to select aspects of care in need of improvement * Comparison of assessment scores to standards in a meeting with a trained peer; identification of personal improvement goals * Program of self-directed learning via 7 small-group meetings with fellow GPs led by trained GP tutors	* Total costs were €117.56 per hour or €2700 per participant * Video assessment was appreciated more than knowledge tests * Written feedback was appreciated; oral feedback from trained peer contributed little * Role of the tutor in group sessions was described as "invaluable"

continued

TABLE A-2 Continued

Reference	Study Purpose	Sample, Method, Outcome Measures, and Duration
Lagerløv, P., M. Loeb, M. Andrew, and P. Hjortdahl. 2000. Improving doctors' prescribing behaviour through reflection on guidelines and prescription feedback: A randomised controlled study. *International Journal for Quality in Health Care* 9(3):159-165.	Study the effect on the quality of prescribing by a combined intervention of providing individual feedback and deriving quality criteria using guideline recommendations by peer review groups	**Sample:** 199 GPs in Norway **Method:** Randomized controlled trial • Experimental group: focus on urinary tract infection (and vice versa) • Control group: focus on asthma **Outcome measures:** Difference in prescribing behavior between the year before and the year after the intervention; self-report of intent to change disease management approach **Duration:** 21 months
Laprise, R. J., R. Thivierge, G. Gosselin, M. Bujas-Bobanovic, S. Vandal, D. Paquette, M. Luneau, P. Julien, S. Goulet, J. Desaulniers, and P. Maltais. 2009. Improved cardiovascular prevention using best CME practices: A randomized trial. *Journal of Continuing Education in the Health Professions* 29(1):16-31.	Determine if after a CME event, practice enablers and reinforcers addressing clinical barriers to preventive care would be more effective in improving adherence to cardiovascular guidelines than a CME event alone	**Sample:** 122 GPs **Method:** Cluster randomized trial • Experimental group: CME event followed by practice enablers and reinforcers • Control group: CME event alone **Outcome measures:** Proportion of patients undermanaged at baseline who received preventive care action

Description of Educational Method	Findings
* Participation in 2 peer meetings to discuss treatment guidelines and agree on common quality criteria for prescribing * Prescription feedback provided to each GP	* Improved prescribing behavior in accordance with guideline recommendations * Group discussion and feedback were well regarded by participants
Nurses visited GPs' offices once a month to • Screen medical records for high-risk patients • Prompt physicians to reassess preventive care of these patients • Enclose a checklist in the patient chart with guideline reminders	Practice enablers and reinforcers following CME significantly improved adherence to guidelines compared to CME alone (OR = 1.78; 95% CI: 1.32-2.41)

continued

TABLE A-2 Continued

Reference	Study Purpose	Sample, Method, Outcome Measures, and Duration
Martin, C. M., G. S. Doig, D. K. Heyland, T. Morrison, and W. J. Sibbald. 2004. Multicentre, cluster-randomized clinical trial of algorithms for critical-care enteral and parenteral therapy (ACCEPT). *Canadian Medical Association Journal* 170(2):197-204.	Test the hypothesis that evidence-based algorithms to improve nutritional support in the intensive care unit (ICU) would improve patient outcomes	**Sample:** 499 patients in 14 ICUs over an 11-month period **Method:** Cluster randomized controlled trial • Experimental group: introduction of evidence-based recommendations • Control group: no intervention **Outcome measures:** Days of enteral nutrition, length of stay in hospital, mortality rates, length of stay in ICU **Duration:** 11 months
Monaghan, M. S., P. D. Turner, M. Z. Skrabal, and R. M. Jones. 2000. Evaluating the format and effectiveness of a disease state management training program for diabetes. *American Journal of Pharmaceutical Education* 64(2):181-184.	Determine whether a CE approach to disease management training in diabetes mellitus is an effective means of improving both cognitive knowledge and confidence levels of participants	**Sample:** 25 pharmacists participating in a training program **Method:** Cohort study with pre- and post-intervention design **Outcome measures:** Scores on a pre- and post-test examination; scores on a 15-item attitudinal questionnaire **Duration:** 14 months

Description of Educational Method	Findings
Evidence-based recommendations were introduced via in-service education sessions, reminders by a local dietitian, posters, and academic detailing	* Patients in intervention ICUs received significantly more days of enteral nutrition (6.7 vs. 5.4 per 10 patient-days; $p = 0.042$), had a significantly shorter mean stay in hospital (25 vs. 35 days; $p = 0.003$), and showed a trend toward reduced mortality (27% vs. 37%; $p = 0.058$) than patients in control ICUs * Mean stay in the ICU did not differ between control and experimental groups
Traditional lectures and small-group exercises in which participants obtained "hands-on" information related to the pharmacist's role	* Cognitive post-test scores (68.8%) improved significantly ($p < 0.001$) over the pre-test scores (49.6%) * Post-test scores on all 15 attitudinal items significantly improved over pre-test scores ($p < 0.012$)

continued

TABLE A-2 Continued

Reference	Study Purpose	Sample, Method, Outcome Measures, and Duration
Naunton, M., G. M. Peterson, G. Jones, G. M. Griffin, and M. D. Bleasel. 2004. Multifaceted educational program increases prescribing of preventive medication for corticosteroid induced osteoporosis. *Journal of Rheumatology* 31(3):550-556.	Assess a comprehensive educational program aimed at increasing the use of osteoporosis preventive therapy in patients prescribed long-term oral corticosteroids	**Sample:** All patients admitted to the Royal Hobart Hospital, Australia; all physicians and pharmacists in 2 regions in Australia **Method:** Controlled trial • Experimental group: geographic region received multifaceted educational program • Control group: geographic region received no intervention **Outcome measures:** Evaluation feedback from GPs and pharmacists; drug utilization data **Duration:** 17 months
Pronovost, P. J., S. M. Berenholtz, C. Goeschel, I. Thom, S. R. Watson, C. G. Holzmueller, J. S. Lyon, L. H. Lubomski, D. A. Thompson, D. Needham, R. Hyzy, R. Welsh, G. Roth, J. Bander, L. Morlock, and J. B. Sexton. 2008. Improving patient safety in intensive care units in Michigan. *Journal of Critical Care* 23(2):207-221.	Describe the design and lessons learned from implementing a large-scale patient safety collaborative and the impact of an intervention on teamwork climate in intensive care units	**Sample:** 99 ICUs across the state of Michigan over 24 months **Method:** Cohort study of ICU teams **Outcome measures:** Improvements in safety culture scores using a teamwork questionnaire; adherence to evidence-based interventions for ventilated patients **Duration:** 17 months

Description of Educational Method	Findings
All GPs and pharmacies in the study area were sent educational materials and guidelines; received academic detailing visits and reminders; and were provided educational magnets for their patients	* Use of preventive therapy increased from 31% of admitted hospital patients taking corticosteroids to 57% post-intervention ($p < 0.0001$) * Significant increase in the use of preventive therapy in the intervention region over the control region ($p < 0.01$)
* Collaborative project included group meetings and conference calls to share best practices and evaluate performance * Partnership between hospital leadership, ICU improvement teams, and ICU staff to identify and resolve barriers * Daily goals communication toolkits for staff education, redesign of work processes, and support of local opinion leaders	* Teamwork climate improved from baseline to post-intervention ($t(71) = -2.921$, $p < 0.005$) * Post-intervention: 46% had >60% consensus of good teamwork; pre-intervention: 17% of ICUs had >60% consensus of good teamwork

continued

TABLE A-2 Continued

Reference	Study Purpose	Sample, Method, Outcome Measures, and Duration
Rashotte, J., M. Thomas, D. Grégoire, and S. Ledoux. 2008. Implementation of a two-part unit-based multiple intervention: Moving evidence-based practice into action. *Canadian Journal of Nursing Research* 40(2):94-114.	Examine the impact and sustained change of a 2-part, unit-based multiple intervention on the use by pediatric critical care nurses of guidelines for pressure-ulcer prevention	**Sample:** 23 pediatric critical care nurses in a Canadian pediatric ICU **Method:** Cohort study **Outcome measures:** Before-and-after measures of frequency of use of interventions as documented in patient records and by observation **Duration:** 6 months
Richards, D., L. Toop, and P. Graham. 2003. Do clinical practice education groups result in sustained change in GP prescribing? *Family Practice* 20(2):199-206.	Determine whether a peer-led small-group educational program is an effective tool in changing practice when added to audit and feedback, academic detailing, and educational bulletins	**Sample:** 230 GPs in urban New Zealand **Method:** Retrospective analysis of a controlled trial • Experimental group: audit and feedback, individual academic detailing, educational bulletins, and peer-led group academic detailing sessions • Control group: audit and feedback, academic detailing, and educational bulletins **Outcome measure:** Targeted prescribing for 12 months before and 24 months after education sessions **Duration:** 36 months

Description of Educational Method	Findings
* Part I targeted individuals with independent and group learning activities: laminated pocket guides, bedside decision-making algorithm * Part II incorporated local and organizational strategies: unit champions, bedside coaching, development of standards	Significant change in implementation of 2 of 11 recommended practices following both interventions ($p < 0.001$)
* Clinical practice education groups met monthly * GP-led discussion of evidence-based topics * Individual prescribing data provided to each GP	* Peer-led small-group discussions had a sustained, positive effect on prescribing behavior that was in addition to any effect of the other educational methods (mean effect size = 1.20) * Mean duration of significant effect was 14.5 months (CI: 95%)

continued

TABLE A-2 Continued

Reference	Study Purpose	Sample, Method, Outcome Measures, and Duration
Saini, B., L. Smith, C. Armour, and I. Krass. 2006. An educational intervention to train community pharmacists in providing specialized asthma care. *American Journal of Pharmaceutical Education* 70(5):118-126.	Test the effect of an educational intervention on pharmacist satisfaction and practice behavior as well as patient outcomes	**Sample:** 27 pharmacists providing asthma care to 102 patients in Australia **Method:** Controlled trial • Experimental group: educational intervention • Control group: no intervention **Outcome measures:** Participant reactions gauged using a questionnaire; asthma severity; peak flow indices; medication costs per patient **Duration:** 6 months
Schneeweiss, S., and S. Ratnapalan. 2007. Impact of a multifaceted pediatric sedation course: Self-directed learning versus a formal continuing medical education course to improve knowledge of sedation guidelines. *Canadian Journal of Emergency Medical Care* 9(2):93-100.	Evaluate the effectiveness of a sedation course in improving physicians' knowledge of pediatric procedural sedation guidelines, relative to self-directed learning	**Sample:** 48 emergency staff physicians, fellows, and residents in a pediatric emergency department **Method:** Randomized controlled trial • Experimental group: self-directed learning • Control group: formal, 4-hour course **Outcome measures:** Scores on multiple choice pre- and post-intervention exam **Duration:** 2 weeks

Description of Educational Method	Findings
Self-directed learning, small-group learning, and workshops with case studies in addition to asthma care training provided in a lecture	* Significant reduction in asthma severity in the experimental group ($p < 0.001$) vs. the control group * In the experimental group, peak flow indices improved from 82.7% at baseline to 87.4% ($p < 0.0010$) at the final visit * Significant reduction in defined daily dose of albuterol used by patients ($p < 0.015$)
* The 4-hour course consisted of small-group and didactic instruction with case studies * The self-directed group received a package with learning objectives, guidelines, a pocket card, and reading materials	Control group's median exam score (83.3%; range: 75.8-96.5%) was significantly higher ($p < 0.0001$) than median exam score of the experimental group (73.3%; range: 43.5-86.6%)

continued

TABLE A-2 Continued

Reference	Study Purpose	Sample, Method, Outcome Measures, and Duration
Scholes, D., L. Grothaus, J. McClure, R. Reid, P. Fishman, C. Sisk, J. E. Lindenbaum, B. Green, J. Grafton, and R. S. Thompson. 2006. A randomized trial of strategies to increase *Chlamydia* screening in young women. *Preventive Medicine* 43(4):343-350.	Evaluate an intervention to increase guideline-recommended *Chlamydia* screening	**Sample:** 23 primary care clinics; 3,509 sexually active females ages 14-25 **Method:** Randomized controlled trial • Experimental group: enhanced guideline intervention • Control group: standard guideline implementation instructions **Outcome measures:** Post-intervention *Chlamydia* testing rates **Duration:** 27 months
Young, J. M., C. D'Este, and J. E. Ward. 2002. Improving family physicians' use of evidence-based smoking cessation strategies: A cluster randomization trial. *Preventive Medicine* 35(6):572-583.	Evaluate a multifaceted, practice-based intervention involving audit, feedback, and academic detailing to improve family physician smoking cessation advice	**Sample:** 60 family physicians in Australia **Method:** Cluster randomized controlled trial • Experimental group: multifaceted intervention • Control group: no intervention **Outcome measures:** Delivery of smoking cessation advice determined by patient recall, physician report, and medical record audit; utilization of nicotine replacement therapies **Duration:** 6 months

NOTE: NA = Not applicable.

Description of Educational Method	Findings
The enhanced guideline group used clinic-based opinion leaders, individual measurement and feedback, exam room reminders, and chart prompts	* Enhanced intervention did not significantly affect *Chlamydia* testing (OR = 1.08; 95% CI: 0.92-1.26; $p = 0.31$) * Testing rates increased among women making preventive care visits in intervention vs. control clinics
* Audit and feedback conducted by a medical peer * Medical record prompt in the form of Post-it notes on medical records * Provision of additional resources for physicians and patients	* Significant increase in the experimental group over the control group in the use of nicotine replacement gum ($p = 0.0002$) and patches ($p = 0.0056$) * No significant differences between groups in smokers' recall or documentation in medical record of specific cessation advice

Appendix B

Health Professions Table

The committee includes the professions listed in Table B-1 in its scope of health professions. The committee reviewed those professions classified by the Bureau of Labor Statistics' *Occupational Outlook Handbook 2008-2009* as "healthcare practitioner and technical occupations," "health technologists and technicians," and "healthcare support occupations." The scope of professions was further defined based on the highest level of formal education—those professions not requiring a baccalaureate or higher degree were not selected and are crossed out in Table B-1.

For each profession that fits within the committee's scope of health professions, Table B-1 also lists the approximate size, average amount of required annual continuing education (CE) credits, and average amount charged per credit. Cost per credit indicates the average amount charged by the major professional society and does not include the costs incurred by employers, private CE providers, or commercial support. It is important to note that the cost per credit ranges dramatically based on CE provider, from being free to costing upwards of $1,000 per course. These data were generally collected through personal communications with professional societies.

TABLE B-1 Health Care Occupations Identified in the Bureau of Labor Statistics' *Occupational Outlook Handbook 2008-2009*

Occupation	Minimum Degree	No. in Profession	Average No. of Credits	Cost per Credit
		Health Care Practitioners and Technical Occupations		
Audiologists	Doctorate	12,826	12.5	$39[a]
Chiropractors	Doctorate	65,000	17	$17
Dentists, General	Doctorate	141,315	18	$28-$42
Oral and Maxillofacial Surgeons	Doctorate	7,044	18	$28-$42
Orthodontists	Doctorate	10,184	18	$28-$42
Prosthodontists	Doctorate	3,404	18	$28-$42
Optometrists	Doctorate	33,000[f]	18	$20-$27
Pharmacists	Doctorate	230,000	15	$30
Physicians and Surgeons	Doctorate	816,727	28	$30
Clinical Psychologist	Master's, Doctorate	39,731	16	$15-$20
Physical Therapists	Master's, Doctorate	175,488	30	$30
Occupational Therapists	Master's	101,560	12	$27.50
Speech-Language Pathologists	Master's	118,270	12.5	$39
Social Workers	Bachelor's, many require Master's	555,000	12.5	$0-$50
Physician Assistants	Bachelor's/PA program	79,980	25	$30
Registered Nurses	Bachelor's, Associate's, or diploma	2,909,357	12	$8-$10

Radiation Therapists	Bachelor's, Associate's with certificate	18,110	12	$8
Dietitians and Nutritionists	Bachelor's	57,000[f]	15	$50
Recreational Therapists	Bachelor's	25,000[f]	10[b]	$17.50-$75
Pathology Assistants	Associate's (NOT IN BLS)	N/A	N/A	N/A
Respiratory Therapists	Associate's	N/A	N/A	N/A
Health Technologists and Technicians				
Medical and Clinical Laboratory Technologists	Bachelor's	167,000[f]	12[c]	$12
Orthotists and Prosthetists	Bachelor's	5,490[f]	18[b]	$7-$15
Occupational Health and Safety Specialists	Bachelor's	45,000[f]	15	$15
Athletic Trainers	Bachelor's	17,000[f]	23[d]	$0-$25
Radiologic Technologists and Technicians	Associate's, certificate, Bachelor's	196,000[f]	11[e]	$8
Surgical Technologists	Certificate, diploma, Associate's	N/A	N/A	N/A
Medical and Clinical Laboratory Technicians	Certificate, diploma, Associate's	N/A	N/A	N/A
Dental Hygienists	Associate's	N/A	N/A	N/A
Cardiovascular Technologists and Technicians	Associate's	N/A	N/A	N/A
Nuclear Medicine Technologists	Certificate, diploma, Associate's	N/A	N/A	N/A

continued

230

TABLE B-1 Continued

Occupation	Minimum Degree	No. in Profession	Average No. of Credits	Cost per Credit
Licensed Practical and Licensed Vocational Nurses	Associate's	N/A	N/A	N/A
Medical Records and Health Information Technicians	Associate's	N/A	N/A	N/A
Occupational Health and Safety Technicians	Certificate, Associate's, Bachelor's, Master's	N/A	N/A	N/A
Dietetic Technicians	Vocational award, Associate's	N/A	N/A	N/A
Psychiatric Technicians	Vocational award	N/A	N/A	N/A
Emergency Medical Technicians and Paramedics	High-school diploma	N/A	N/A	N/A
Opticians, Dispensing	High-school diploma	N/A	N/A	N/A
Diagnostic Medical Sonographers	None	N/A	N/A	N/A
Pharmacy Technicians	None	N/A	N/A	N/A
Health Care Support Occupations				
Occupational Therapist Assistants	Associate's, certificate	N/A	N/A	N/A
Physical Therapist Assistants	High school diploma, Associate's	N/A	N/A	N/A
Medical Assistants	Vocational school (1 or 2 yr)	N/A	N/A	N/A
Medical Transcriptionists	Postsecondary training preferred	N/A	N/A	N/A
Nursing Aides, Orderlies, and Attendants	High-school diploma (aides)	N/A	N/A	N/A

Psychiatric Aides	High school diploma	N/A	N/A	N/A
Dental Assistants	High school diploma	N/A	N/A	N/A
Home Health Aides	None	N/A	N/A	N/A
Occupational Therapist Aides	None	N/A	N/A	N/A
Physical Therapist Aides	None	N/A	N/A	N/A
Massage Therapists	None	N/A	N/A	N/A
Medical Equipment Preparers	None	N/A	N/A	N/A
Pharmacy Aides	None	N/A	N/A	N/A

NOTE: N/A = Not applicable.

[a] This is the average cost of an American Speech-Language-Hearing Association Professional Development distance learning program.

[b] For national certification.

[c] Only 12 states and Puerto Rico require licensure (CA, GA, HI, FL, LA, MT, ND, NV, NY, RI, TN, WV).

[d] Only 32 states require continuing education credits.

[e] Only 28 states require continuing education credits.

[f] Data from Bureau of Labor Statistics.

Appendix C

International Comparison of Continuing Education and Continuing Professional Development

Examining international models and trends in continuing education (CE) and continuing professional development (CPD) for health professionals has been, and continues to be, an area of interest for the global community of health professionals and education theorists. A 1999 report prepared for the Organisation for Economic Co-operation and Development (OECD) emphasizes the importance of internationally comparable data for advancing the study of CE. Cross-fertilization of innovative education models provides comparative formative and summative evaluations to validate and improve best practices while leading the way toward international coherence on the training, registration, and continual assessment of health professionals (Merkur et al., 2008b).

This comparative synthesis, which primarily includes examples from Canada, Australia, the United Kingdom, and other European countries,[1] reviews the development of and current practices in medical, nursing, dental, and pharmacy CE and CPD. The paucity of descriptive literature available made it necessary to limit this review to these selected professions.

This review aims to address three questions:

1. Do definitions and mechanisms of CE and CPD differ, and to what extent are they tied to revalidation and licensure?

---

[1] For the purposes of this review, the United Kingdom is examined separately from the rest of Europe.

2. Have countries changed or adapted their CE or CPD systems to improve content or learning methods, and how have they dealt with pharmaceutical support for CE?
3. What can the United States learn from the experiences of other countries?

The literature search, performed in December 2008, included the EBSCO, OVID, Academic Search Premier, and Medline databases. Keywords included continuing professional development, European learning, international, continuing education, nursing, pharmacy, medicine/medical, dental/dentistry, accreditation, revalidation, and competence. This review indicates requirements for training, types of training, and the mechanisms by which the requirements are enforced. However, much about the effectiveness of many of these models remains unknown.

The diverse definitions and terminologies associated with CE and CPD systems complicate comparative analyses. While CE credits or hours are the currency by which regulatory bodies often assess competence, these regulatory bodies have a myriad of purposes and synonyms, including licensure, certification, credentialing, and revalidation. For example, Merkur and colleagues (2008a) define revalidation as aiming to "demonstrate that the competence of doctors is acceptable." These regulatory processes may include periodic application forms, fees, and required participation in activities, such as CE, CPD, and peer assessment, to maintain and improve competence.

Just as CE requirements within professions vary by state in the United States, Canadian licensing bodies, for example, which differ between jurisdictions of practice (i.e., provinces, territories), do not agree on requirements for CE and CPD as part of their processes for ensuring the competence of health professionals. The degree of inclusion of CE credits in revalidation and relicensure systems varies between and within countries.

In the early 1990s, Australia, Canada, and the United Kingdom gradually shifted from CE to CPD. Whereas CE serves to update and reinforce knowledge (e.g., management of heart attacks, how to diagnose HIV), CPD deals with personal, communication, managerial, and team-building skills in addition to content (Merkur et al., 2008a; Peck et al., 2000). Limitations in the traditional methods of CE (e.g., educational courses, lectures) led to the development of the more self-directed and self-reflective approach, which is believed to encourage lifelong learning and better meet the educational needs of health professionals (Evans et al., 2002). For example, in 1997 the government of the United Kingdom stressed the role of CPD in ensuring quality and encouraged professional bodies to strengthen systems for self-regulation and lifelong learning (UK Department of Health, 1997). This process of CPD, defined by Davis and colleagues as an "umbrella for all sorts of interventions," including CE, ties learning more closely to practice (Davis et al., 2003, p. 11). Compared to CE, which is frequently based on acquiring credits, CPD relies on processes of self-accreditation and reflection via personal portfolios.

COMPARATIVE EXAMPLES OF CONTINUING MEDICAL EDUCATION

In a series of articles in the *British Medical Journal* exploring how the United States can improve its health care system, Quam and Smith (2005) argue the United States could improve its continuing medical education (CME) system by more closely mirroring the United Kingdom's guidelines for CPD. A brief historical survey provides the background in which CE systems can adapt and change based on international models presented in Table C-1.

Although methods of CE are continually evolving around the world, CE models may be classified into two distinct categories: the learning model, seeking to improve clinical competence, and the assessment model that emphasizes both performance and competence (Merkur et al., 2008a). These CE models are presented in Table C-2. The majority of countries use the learning model only. While some countries (e.g., Austria, France, the Netherlands, United Kingdom) screen all physicians for competence, no countries included in the 2008 comparative survey used more selected, targeted screenings to ensure competence.

Maintenance of Certification in Canada

Through the latter half of the twentieth century, Canadian concepts of CME developed alongside those in the United States until patient advocacy, government regulation, and an increase in medical knowledge led the Royal College of Physicians and Surgeons of Canada (RCPSC) to explore new frameworks for continued competency. The framework, known as CanMEDS, was adopted in 1996 and outlines essential physician competencies with the aim of improving patient care. A program of mandatory professional development, called the Maintenance of Certification (MOC) program was mandated by the RCPSC beginning in 2000 (Royal College of Physicians and Surgeons of Canada, 2008). At this time, fellows of the college

TABLE C-1 Continuing Medical Education—An International
Comparison

| Country | Ways of Ensuring Competence | | |
	CME or CPD	Peer Review	Compulsory
Australia	CPD	No	No
Austria	CME	Yes	Yes
Belgium	CME & CPD	Yes	No
Canada	CPD	Yes	No
France	CME	Yes	Yes
Germany	CME	No	Yes for government employees

Incentives			
+	–	Regulating Authority	Requirements
	Financial disincentives for noncompliance	Respective medical colleges and faculties (professional bodies)	Cycle varies between 3 and 5 years. Mandatory components vary by college
	Legal requirement	Austrian Medical Chamber (professional body)	150 1-hour credits over 3 years
Financial incentive (4% salary increase)		Minister of Public Health (government body)	20 hours every year OR accreditation (requires 200 credit hours over 3 years and participation in two peer reviews per year)
Participation awards		Royal College of Physicians and Surgeons (professional body)	400 credits over 5 years (some activities worth more credits based on content)
	Lawsuits by regional councils	National Councils for Continuing Medical Education (professional bodies)	
	Reduced reimbursement; accreditation withdrawn	Regional chambers of physicians (professional bodies)	250 45-minute credits over 5 years

continued

TABLE C-1 Continued

Country	Ways of Ensuring Competence		
	CME or CPD	Peer Review	Compulsory
Italy	CPD	No	Yes
The Netherlands	CME & CPD	Yes for specialists	Yes
New Zealand	CPD	No	Yes
Spain	CME (9 of 17 regions)	No	No
United Kingdom	CPD	Yes: 360° feedback[a]	Pending
United States	CME	No	Yes

NOTE: CME = continuing medical education; CPD = continuing professional development.

[a] 360° feedback is a process whereby colleagues (including nursing and administrative staff) evaluate a physician's performance. The process was initially developed in the commercial sector as a means of highlighting an employee's strengths as well as areas in need of improvement.

SOURCES: Merkur et al., 2008a,b; Peck et al., 2000.

Incentives			
+	−	Regulating Authority	Requirements
None		Continuing Medical Education Commission of the Ministry of Health (government body)	150 1-hour credits over 5 years
	Removal from medical registry	Committees of specialists and primary care physicians (professional body)	200 hours of credits over 5 years; peer visitation every 5 years (only for specialists)
	Forced work supervision; loss of registration	Medical colleges and faculties (professional bodies)	Variable by region and college
Variable by region		Spanish Medical Association (professional body)	Variable by region
	Forced work supervision	Department of Health (government)	Parallel requirements: (1) relicensure every 5 years and (2) recertification (variable by college)
Variable by state			Variable by state

TABLE C-2 Synthesis of Models for Assessing Continuing Competence

Models for Assessing Continuing Competence	Pros	Cons	Countries Using the Model
Learning Model: CE seeks to improve clinical competence	Seeks to improve clinical competence	Does not identify poorly performing professionals	Australia Austria Belgium Canada France Germany Italy The Netherlands New Zealand Spain United Kingdom United States
Assessment Model: emphasizes both performance and competence *Responsive Assessment:* assessment when a complaint or problem occurs	Potential to identify poor performers	Cannot identify all poorly performing professionals and requires centralized complaint system	None
Periodic Assessment: full assessment of all domains of competence for all physicians	Potential to identify poor performers	Very ambitious and potentially unfeasible	None

241

Screening Assessment for All: identifies incompetence using peer review and patient questionnaires	Potential to identify poor performers	No single screening test has been developed that reliably and practically indicates poor performance	Austria France Hungary Ireland The Netherlands Slovenia United Kingdom
Screening Assessment for High-Risk Groups: assesses poorly performing professionals (e.g., based on patient outcomes or prescribing patterns) or targeting groups using other known qualities (i.e., older doctors)	Potential to identify poor performers	May contravene privacy laws and requires a database of physician performance measures	None

SOURCE: Merkur et al, 2008a.

(approximately 90 percent of certified physicians in Canada are fellows of the RCPSC) were mandated to assess their professional needs and record participation in CPD, as well as learning outcomes achieved for their practice. The MOC program aims to make CPD an educational initiative to improve practice as opposed to an administrative burden (Campbell, 2008). Box C-1 describes how technology is used to decrease the administrative burden placed on health professionals.

Maintenance of Professional Standards in Australia and New Zealand

In 1994, alongside Canada, the Royal Australasian College of Physicians (RACP)[2] broke ground in CME by implementing a strategy to promote CPD. This CPD scheme, known as the Maintenance of Professional Standards (MOPS) program, included the accumulation of credit points and the recording of those points in a diary system. In consultation with the Royal College of Physicians and Surgeons of Canada, RACP is now phasing out MOPS and moving toward a fully electronic system. Between May 2008 and 2010, all RACP fellows will transition to an e-folio CPD system. This system will enhance opportunities for prospective learning by facilitating individual CPD plans tailored to individually identified needs and competencies (Royal Australasian College of Physicians, 2008).

Continuing Professional Development in the United Kingdom

While participation in CPD has long been a condition of employment in the National Health Service (NHS), a string of unfortunate, and perhaps preventable, incidents spurred changes in the United Kingdom's CPD system (Wall and Halligan, 2006). Most notably, a 2001 government inquiry into pediatric cardiac surgeries performed at Bristol Royal Infirmary focused attention on poor clinical teamwork, a severe lack of performance data, and an absence of reflective practice. The government and the public demanded competent health professionals; thus, the CME system in the United Kingdom is composed of three interrelated yet separately monitored and administered parts, each of which requires CPD: (1) mandatory recertification, (2) annual appraisal (for doctors in England), and (3) mandatory revalidation.

---

[2] In Australia, individual medical colleges, of which RACP is one, regulate CME requirements.

BOX C-1
An Integrated System for CE

The College of Family Physicians of Canada (CFPC), which accredits activities in which family physicians participate, has an integrated system for CME, called Maintenance of Proficiency (known as Mainpro). Mainpro is based on the principle that physicians should plan and manage their own programs of self-directed, practice-based, lifelong learning (College of Family Physicians of Canada, 2003). Both the MOC program and Mainpro utilize online tools to aid physicians in tracking their learning objectives and participation in learning events. Individual learning portfolios can be a useful tool for planning and recording learning and incorporating personal development plans. The portfolio can then form the basis for peer or external review, providing documentation necessary for revalidation while also encouraging the individual professional to identify his own learning goals (du Boulay, 2000).

The General Medical Council (GMC) has defined the competencies needed by all doctors, while professional organizations, including for example the Royal College of General Practitioners, have defined the extra competencies needed for their specialties (Quam and Smith, 2005). Like most of the CE systems discussed in this report, the royal college systems depend on the accrual of hours related to credits. To be recertified, a doctor must meet the CPD standards set by his royal college before being said to be "in good standing."

In 2001, the NHS made annual appraisal compulsory for all doctors in England. This process requires the formation of a personal development plan with identified learning needs relevant to the competencies developed by their respective specialist associations. An appraisal process evaluates how the doctor has worked toward meeting those learning needs (Quam and Smith, 2005). This system hinges on the training and competence of its appraisers, all of whom are employed and trained by the NHS.

In 2004, the NHS introduced standards for moving the health care system toward patient-centered care, preventive medicine, and local decision making. Of 37 standards, 3 specifically relate to updating skills and training and participating in peer review and appraisal (UK Department of Health, 2004). The Commission of Healthcare Audit and Inspection has responsibility for the implementation of these standards at an organizational level. In 2008, the Department of Health gave the royal colleges a key role by making the Academy of the Royal Medical Colleges a clearinghouse for funding of

CE development (see Box C-2 for the role of industry funding). For example, "e-Learning for Healthcare" provides cash to individual royal colleges for the development of online learning programs. In sum, the royal colleges develop content, set standards, provide examinations, and accredit the content of events and online courses provided by commercial competitors (Hawkes, 2008).

Disparate Continuing Education Systems in Select European Countries

European countries face a mosaic of CE and CPD stakeholders and incentives for and mechanisms of revalidation (Table C-2). In Belgium, participation in CME yields higher salaries; in the Netherlands, CME is mandatory and failing to participate can result in a physician's removal from the medical registry; and in Italy, mandatory interprofessional training with other professionals such as nurses and medical technicians is the norm (Braido et al., 2005). Professional medical bodies tend to regulate CME in most Western European countries, sometimes within legal frameworks established by national governments; in other countries, however, insurers may require physicians with whom they contract to fulfill specific CME requirements (Merkur et al., 2008a). A patchwork system of funding, including physician self-payment, professional associations or governments subsidizing costs, and pharmaceutical companies contributing to CME, further entangles the CME process.

The European Union, predicated on principles of free movement across borders, has a vested stake in ensuring the mobility of health care professionals. This requires mutual recognition of professional qualifications, but this principle is difficult to uphold because the legal framework in certain countries does not require training beyond initial education whereas other countries make this mandatory. Until 2005, France, for example, did not require any training beyond receipt of a medical diploma. Despite efforts to encourage CE through the use of incentives, physicians did not embrace it; thus, the French government passed a law making CME mandatory. A parallel law made the evaluation of professional practice mandatory for all doctors. While control of these processes was placed under the responsibility of an independent organization, compliance with the requirements is yet unknown (Segouin et al., 2007).

The European Commission [sic] recognized in 2006 the need for minimal standards for CPD for physicians and nurses (European Commission High Level Group on Health Services and Medical Care, 2006). Despite this acknowledgment, a directive was never placed on

---

BOX C-2
The Role of Industry Funding

Despite the differences in CPD and CE, the UK, Canadian, and U.S. systems of CME face similar challenges, one of which is the role of industry-subsidized learning opportunities. A 2008 editorial in the *Canadian Medical Association Journal* called the pharmaceutical industry's role in funding CME in Canada "unacceptable" (Hebert, 2008, p. 179). Although there are no reliable data on the percentage of accredited CME activities in Canada funded by pharmaceutical and medical device manufacturers, there are widely held beliefs that the situation is similar to that in the United States, where $1.21 billion (48 percent of all money spent on accredited CME) in 2007 came from commercial support (ACCME, 2008; Spurgeon, 2008). For example, while online CME is an important approach to CPD in Canada, much online CME is currently funded directly or indirectly by industry. As a result, in January 2008, the Canadian Medical Association convened a meeting of national specialty societies and related medical organizations to discuss issues related to online CME, particularly how the sources of funding might be identified.

A study published in 2003 by a team of Scottish researchers found that the pharmaceutical industry funded approximately half of CME in the United Kingdom. Since that time, the Association of the British Pharmaceutical Industry has introduced a code of conduct, including a ban on gifts worth more than 6 pounds sterling and a guideline that companies do not pay for "key opinion leaders" to attend conferences abroad (Hawkes, 2008).

Because pharmaceutical companies, in particular, generally target prescribers as their clients, conflicted funding sources are not nearly as prominent an issue in CE for nurses, dentists, and pharmacists as they are for physicians.

---

the agenda to develop these standards. Harmonized systems of CME still need to be developed, potentially by the European Accreditation Council for Continuing Medical Education (Braido et al., 2005).

COMPARATIVE EXAMPLES OF
CONTINUING NURSING EDUCATION

A systematic review of nursing education and regulation stresses the importance of Europe's harmonizing nursing education systems to minimize problems with nursing retention and recruitment (Robinson and Griffiths, 2007). The review of 18 countries including the United States acknowledges difficulties in obtaining accurate information on CE requirements for nurses and documents disparate examples of nursing CE systems.

The United Kingdom, which has acknowledged the need for a functioning system of CE for nurses since the mid-1990s (Nolan et al., 1995), has a system in which nurses must register with the Nursing and Midwifery Council. This registration requires triannual renewal dependent on evidence that CPD was performed. Similarly, advanced degree nurses in Japan (as categorized by their level of education) must apply for certificate renewal every 5 years, a process requiring participation in designated CPD events and the development of a practice report. Nurses with advanced degrees (postbaccalaurate) do not, however, need to renew their certifications or engage in CE (Harayama, 1994).

To further illustrate the vast differences that exist in nursing regulation, licensure, and CE, Swedish nurses must register with the National Board of Health and Welfare but are not regulated once licensed (Josefsson et al., 2008). In Denmark, to deal with specific local education needs, the Branch Boards of the Denmark Nursing Organisation offers study days and seminars on topical issues (Vejlgaard, 2003). Similarly, Italian universities, health care institutions, and CE agencies offer courses for speciality nurses, allowing them to choose among relevant training (Robinson and Griffiths, 2007).

COMPARATIVE EXAMPLES OF
CONTINUING DENTAL EDUCATION

In order to build a culture of professional competency, the Association for Dental Education in Europe (ADEE), an organization that promotes high standards of dental education to its membership of European dental schools, specialist societies, and national dental bodies, has emphasized that undergraduate education should "act as a springboard which engenders the concept of continuing professional development and life long learning" (Cowpe et al., 2008, p. 20). In its *Profile and Competencies for the European Dentist* (2008), the ADEE states that upon graduation, a dentist must seek CE on an annual basis and demonstrate this through the use of a logbook or e-folio. Additionally, graduating dentists must prove competency in using information technology for documentation of participation in CE.

The Commonwealth Dental Association, a trade association comprised of 53 countries currently or formerly associated with the British crown, conducted a review of its dental workforce in 2007. Mandatory CE for dentists was limited to eight of the surveyed nations, including Canada, New Zealand, the United Kingdom, and the Victoria region of Australia (Table C-3). Of these, only New

TABLE C-3 Continuing Dental Education—An International Comparison

	Compulsory	Requirements
Australia	No, except in one state (Victoria)	Unknown
Canada	Yes	Variable by province
New Zealand	Yes	160 hours over 4 years
United Kingdom	Yes	75 hours of formal courses and 250 hours of nonformal education over 5 years
United States	Yes (in 49 states)	Variable by state

SOURCE: Kravitz, 2007.

Zealand and the United Kingdom have countrywide mandates for CE for dentists.

The United Kingdom's General Dental Council instituted its CE program in 2002, preceeding New Zealand's countrywide CE program for dentists by 12 months. In addition to completing CE courses, all dentists contracted with the NHS must complete 15 hours of peer review every 3 years. A systematic survey of 2,082 dentists in three regions of England examined the effectiveness of the NHS mandate for CE for dentists based on the frequency and types of CE activities in which a dentist participated (Bullock et al., 2003). The review concluded that dentists have little personal incentive to engage in activities other than CE courses and discussion with colleagues because the mandate permits dentists to choose the methods of CE activities in which they engage and does not, for example, require peer review. Mandated professional development plans are one means of reflection and thus may be an appropriate vehicles of CE for dentists.

COMPARATIVE EXAMPLES OF CONTINUING PHARMACEUTICAL EDUCATION

A report prepared for the International Pharmaceutical Foundation (FIP) acknowledges a breadth of new knowledge relevant to the field of pharmacy and the important role CE plays in maintaining and updating pharmaceutical skills and knowledge (International Pharmaceutical Federation, 2006). The FIP initially stressed the link between the development of pharmacy skills and quality improvement when, in 2001, it established the International Forum for Quality Assurance of Pharmacy Education to develop a set of principles for CE programs (Rouse, 2008). Furthermore, the FIP's *Statement of Professional Standards on Continuing Professional Development* includes a provision about a pharmacist's individual responsibility to ensure his own competency through "systematic maintenance, development, and broadening of knowledge, skills, and attitudes" (International Pharmaceutical Federation, 2002). The FIP differentiates CPD from CE by stressing that CPD requires pharmacists to take personal responsibility for planning for their own development, meeting these needs, and subsequently evaluating their success in doing so.

The Pharmacy Workforce Survey, administered in 2005, surveyed 37 countries representing each of the six World Health Organization regions: 9 of the 37 countries had mandatory CE for individual pharmacists (International Pharmaceutical Federation, 2006). Information on the regulatory boards and the CE systems is presented in Table C-4. CE courses for pharmacists, provided by professional associations, pharmacy boards, universities, teaching hospitals, and pharmaceutical companies, vary widely in their scope and breadth of content, and only a few countries (e.g. France, Iraq, Japan, Kenya, Singapore, Zambia) have mandatory accreditation of providers of CE for pharmacists.

APPLICABLE LESSONS FOR THE UNITED STATES

CE, which serves a variety of purposes, may improve quality of care and patient safety while minimizing risks and containing costs. The notion that the acquisition of a qualification is an adequate measure of lifelong competence (Merkur et al., 2008b) has been challenged in recent decades. As a result, many countries are in the process of reforming their CE systems (Braido et al., 2005). Overall, this literature review suggests that the definitions and mechanisms of ensuring competence vary significantly across countries. While divergence exists in monitoring and enforcement, similarities exist as well: most systems rely on professional self-regulation (Peck et al., 2000); a principal barrier for improving and implementing CE systems at the organizational level is lack of financial resources (Merkur et al., 2008a); and the most demanding systems incorporate peer review or practice audit. Although no CE system is obviously superior, considerable scope exists to learn from experiences in other countries.

Increasingly, professional associations and regulatory bodies encourage health professionals to learn together with other professional groups. As an example, health professionals in Italy engage

TABLE C-4 Continuing Pharmaceutical Education—An International Comparison

		Incentives			
	Compulsory	+	–	Regulating Authority	Requirements
Canada	Yes (in most provinces)		Potential for refusal to renew license	Provincial pharmacy boards	Variable by province
France	Yes	Certificate for completion		Ordre National des Pharmaciens and the Social Affairs Ministry	Currently being considered
Germany	No (ethical obligation stated in law)	Certificate for completion		N/A	150 45-minute credits over 3 years
United Kingdom	Yes		Potential for removal from pharmacy register	Pharmacy profession (subnational pharmaceutical associations)	CPD not measured (guidelines advise one CPD entry per month)
United States	Yes		Potential for license revocation	State boards of pharmacy	Most common (varies by state) is 30 hours over 2 years

NOTE: N/A = not applicable.
SOURCE: International Pharmaceutical Federation, 2006.

in interprofessional CE in a system that aims to ensure the impact of education on practice quality (Braido et al., 2005). The Learning Opportunities for Teams (LOTUS) program, facilitated by the European Commission, furthered the advancement of Italy's team-based CE by linking 214 primary care professionals at four sites across Europe. This pilot program, which began in 1997 and has now ended, highlighted the relevance of multidisciplinary facilitation and technology for organizational and individual growth (Mathers et al., 2007). Furthermore, Canada's well-established system of interprofessional education serves as a model for the further development of interprofessional education (Ho et al., 2008) and has recently been adopted by the Royal Dutch Medical Association (Wigersma et al., 2009).

The 2005 examination of CE by the *British Medical Journal* acknowledges widespread acceptance that systems to ensure competence should be nonpunitive, with efforts focused on professional development (Kmietowicz, 2005). Professional organizations could take the lead in this by introducing a system rewarding physicians who participate in CE and CPD. The United States has the opportunity to understand the current challenges in CE both nationally and internationally and to use the platform of CPD as a means to address deficiencies in the current CE system. International CE and CPD systems are vehicles from which the United States can learn, gleaning best practices and offering solutions and leadership.

REFERENCES

ACCME (Accreditation Council for Continuing Medical Education). 2008. *ACCME annual report data 2007*. http://www.accme.org/dir_docs/doc_upload/207fa8e2-bdbe-47f8-9b65-52477f9faade_uploaddocument.pdf (accessed January 16, 2009).

Braido, F., T. Popov, I. J. Ansotegui, J. Gayraud, K. L. Nekam, J. L. Delgado, H. J. Mailing, S. Olson, M. Larche, A. Negri, and G. W. Canonica. 2005. Continuing medical education: An international reality. *Allergy: European Journal of Allergy and Clinical Immunology* 60(6):739-742.

Bullock, A., V. Firmstone, A. Fielding, J. Frame, D. Thomas, and C. Belfield. 2003. Participation of UK dentists in continuing professional development. *British Dental Journal* 194(1):47-51.

Campbell, C. 2008. *Maintenance of certification: Back to the future*. http://rcpsc.medical.org/news/documents/MOCCraig_e.pdf (accessed December 15, 2008).

College of Family Physicians of Canada. 2003. *Mainpro background information*. http://www.cfpc.ca/English/cfpc/cme/mainpro/ (accessed January 23, 2009).

Cowpe, J., A. Plasschaert, W. Harzer, H. Vinkka-Puhakka, and A. D. Walmsley. 2008. *Profile and competencies for the European dentist, update 2008*. Dublin, Ireland: Association for Dental Education in Europe.

Davis, D., B. E. Barnes, and R. D. Fox, eds. 2003. *The continuing professional development of physicians: From research to practice.* Chicago, IL: American Medical Association.

du Boulay, C. 2000. From CME to CPD: Getting better at getting better? *British Medical Journal* 320:393-394.

European Commission High Level Group on Health Services and Medical Care. 2006. *Report on the work of the high level group in 2006.* HLG/2006/8 FINAL European Commission Health and Consumer Protection Directorate-General.

Evans, A., S. Ali, C. Singleton, P. Nolan, and J. Bahrami. 2002. The effectiveness of personal education plans in continuing professional development: An evaluation. *Medical Teacher* 24(1):79-84.

Harayama, T. 1994. Professional socialization of nurses: A comparative study of France and Japan. Paper presented at the 13th World Congress of Sociology, Bielefeld, Germany.

Hawkes, N. 2008. What price education? *British Medical Journal* 337:1080-1081.

Hebert, P. C. 2008. The need for an institute of continuing health education. *Canadian Medical Association Journal* 178(7):805-806.

Ho, K., S. Jarvis-Selinger, F. Borduas, B. Frank, P. Hall, R. Handfield-Jones, D. F. Hardwick, J. Lockyer, D. Sinclair, H. N. Lauscher, L. Ferdinands, A. MacLeod, M. A. Robitaille, and M. Rouleau. 2008. Making interprofessional education work: The strategic roles of the academy. *Academic Medicine* 83(10):934-940.

International Pharmaceutical Federation. 2002. FIP statement of professional standards: Continuing professional development. The Hague, The Netherlands: International Pharmaceutical Federation.

———. 2006. *Global pharmacy workforce and migration report: A call for action.* The Hague, The Netherlands: International Pharmaceutical Federation.

Josefsson, K., L. Sonde, and T. B. Robins Wahlin. 2008. Competence development of registered nurses in municipal elderly care in Sweden: A questionnaire survey. *International Journal of Nursing Studies* 45(3):428-441.

Kmietowicz, Z. 2005. Revalidation must serve doctors and the public. *British Medical Journal* 330(7502):1229.

Kravitz, A. S. 2007. *Survey of the dental workforce in the Commonwealth.* Commonwealth Dental Association.

Mathers, N., G. Maso, J. Heyrman, and O. S. Gaspar. 2007. LOTUS: An evaluation of a European continuing professional development programme. *Education for Primary Care* 18(3):328-337.

Merkur, S., P. Mladovsky, E. Mossialos, and M. McKee. 2008a. *Do lifelong learning and revalidation ensure that physicians are fit to practice?* Paper presented at WHO European Ministerial Conference on Health Systems, Tallin, Estonia, June 25-27.

Merkur, S., E. Mossialos, M. Long, and M. McKee. 2008b. Physician revalidation in Europe. *Clinical Medicine, Journal of the Royal College of Physicians of London* 8(4):371-376.

Nolan, M., R. G. Owens, and J. Nolan. 1995. Continuing professional education: Identifying the characteristics of an effective system. *Journal of Advanced Nursing* 21(3):551-560.

Peck, C., M. McCall, B. McLaren, and T. Rotem. 2000. Continuing medical education and continuing professional development: International comparisons. *British Medical Journal* 320(7232):432-435.

Quam, L., and R. Smith. 2005. US and UK health care: A special relationship? What can the UK and US health systems learn from each other? *British Medical Journal* 330(7490):530-533.

Robinson, S., and P. Griffiths. 2007. *Nursing education and regulation: International profiles and perspectives.* London, UK: National Nursing Research Unit, King's College.

Rouse, M. J. 2008. *A global framework for quality assurance of pharmacy education.* The Hague, The Netherlands: International Forum for Quality Assurance of Pharmacy Education.

Royal Australasian College of Physicians. 2008. *Continuing professional development.* http://www.racp.edu.au/index.cfm?objectid=49F20A15-2A57-5487-D079C4F1E6619D0A (accessed December 16, 2008).

Royal College of Physicians and Surgeons of Canada. 2008. *Maintenance of certification program.* http://rcpsc.medical.org/opd/moc-program/index.php (accessed January 23, 2009).

Segouin, C., J. Jouquan, B. Hodges, P. Brechat, S. David, D. Maillard, B. Schlemmer, and D. Bertrand. 2007. Country report: Medical education in France. *Medical Education* 41:295-301.

Spurgeon, D. 2008. Continuing education should no longer be funded by drug industry, says CMAJ. *British Medical Journal* 336:742-743.

UK Department of Health. 1997. *The new NHS: Modern and dependable.* http://www.archive.official-documents.co.uk/document/doh/newnhs/newnhs.htm (accessed January 26, 2009).

———. 2004. *National standards, local action: Health and social care standards and planning framework, 2005/06-2007/08.* ROCR Ref: 3533. UK Department of Health.

Vejlgaard, T. B. 2003. Educational needs of doctors and nurses working in palliative care. *Ugeskr Laeger* 165(36):3413-3417.

Wall, D., and A. Halligan. 2006. The role of clinical governance in CPD. *European Clinics in Obstetrics and Gynaecology* 1(4):231-240.

Wigersma, L., M. Wesseling, and M. Babovic. 2009. Duidelijk deskundig. Medisch kwaliteitsbeleid moet samenhangender en transparanter. *Medisch Contact* 64:378-381.

Appendix D

Continuing Education in
Professional Fields
Outside of Health Care

Ongoing professional training is part of the development of high quality professionals and is necessary for complex technical professions. To understand the challenges and opportunities facing continuing education (CE) in the health professions, it may be useful to examine professional development activities in other fields. Accountants, engineers, lawyers, commercial pilots, teachers, and the workforces of many other fields also have an ongoing need to improve their skills and stay competent to perform at high levels, spurring the advancement of continuing education activities in these fields. Some are more advanced in CE while others are in their infancy. Although the content of CE in these fields may be quite different from CE in the health professions, their efforts can provide useful and instructive perspectives on CE for health care.

In fields outside of the health professions, "professional development" is commonly used as a term to encompass activities analogous to CE. However, it is important to recognize that professional development is commonly defined as the entire process by which professionals learn and maintain their competence (e.g., undergraduate and graduate school), whereas CE is limited to the sum of the training activities a professional has taken part in over the course of his career.

This appendix reviews the professional development of select professions. The health professions can glean many lessons from other professions, as well as share their best practices. In particular, the ways in which CE is regulated, conducted, and financed are examined.

CONTINUING EDUCATION FOR ACCOUNTANTS

Certified public accountants (CPAs) are, by virtue of their title, certified and licensed by state boards of accountancy. After initial certification, CPAs in 52 of 54 U.S. jurisdictions must meet continuing professional education (CPE) requirements to maintain their licenses.[1] To provide a uniform approach to regulating the accounting profession, the American Institute of Certified Public Accountants (AICPA) and the National Association of State Boards of Accountancy (NASBA) publish Uniform Accountability Act rules that include a requirement for 120 hours of CPE every 3 years (AICPA and NASBA, 2007). Although each state determines its own CPE requirements, all jurisdictions require either 40 hours each year, 80 hours each 2-year period, or 120 hours each 3-year period, with a minimum of 20 hours in each year (VanZante and Fritzsch, 2006).

Methods of CPE for CPAs are generally limited to self-study, either interactive (e.g., CD-ROM programs, web-based self-study) or noninteractive (e.g., journal reading), or live activities ranging from webinars to lectures and conferences. The National Registry of Continuing Professional Education Sponsors recognizes CPE providers that offer programs in accordance with nationally recognized standards (NASBA, 2009), while individual state boards of accountancy recognize providers from which CPAs can receive CPE credits for license renewal.

Recent accounting scandals have highlighted the importance of ethics in accounting (Mele, 2005). In line with this, some states, including New York and Texas, require CPAs to take some level of CPE related to ethics. Other states have specific requirements for individuals who perform tasks such as attest or auditing services (VanZante and Fritzsch, 2006), and the federal government has content-specific standards for CPAs' performing auditing work (GAO, 2005). The price of courses and webinars, among others, generally varies based on the technicality of the program's content, the number of credit hours earned, and the provider. A typical 8-hour course offered by a professional association (e.g., Pennsylvania Institute of CPAs, California Society of CPAs) averages between $200 and $300, while a 1-hour webinar generally costs between $40 and $100.

---

[1] Wisconsin and the U.S. Virgin Islands do not have CE requirements for license renewal (VanZante and Fritzsch, 2006).

For CPAs in many national firms or working in business or industry, the costs of CPE are usually borne by the CPA's employer, whereas some solo practitioners and some employees of local and regional firms pay for CPE out of pocket.[2]

The AICPA-NASBA Uniform Accountability Act also stipulates that CPAs are not required to submit documentation of every CPE course they have attended; rather, they are required to sign a statement indicating their compliance with state requirements (AICPA and NASBA, 2007). Some states have instituted random verification to ensure compliance; the Pennsylvania State Board of Accountancy, for example, verifies 10 percent of renewal applications.

CONTINUING EDUCATION FOR ENGINEERS

With a need for lifelong education to stay up to date in the many rapidly evolving fields of engineering, CE is becoming an increasingly important, standardized method of ensuring professional competence. CE in engineering resembles CE in the health professions both in the formats through which it is offered and in the overall goal of competence. The National Council of Examiners for Engineering and Surveying (NCEES) uses the term "continuing professional competency" to discuss CE.

Although continuing professional competency requirements are mandated at the state level, as of June 2008, NCEES requires at least 15 professional development hours per year for licensure (NCEES, 2008). In engineering, professional development hours are the common currency for CE (continuing education units are also used but refer only to continuing education and training). Licensure requirements vary by state, type of engineering, and licensing body and therefore do not follow a uniform standard. However, licensure is not necessary for practice but may be required for certain jobs and areas of engineering. State requirements vary from no mandatory CE hours to 20 mandatory CE hours per year to maintain licensure (CSI Construction Education Network, 2008). Certification is awarded by area of engineering and generally needs to be continuously updated.

Professional development hours can be earned by successful completion of college or continuing education courses, completing short courses or tutorials such as those offered by distance education, giving presentations at meetings or workshops, teaching or

---

[2] Personal communication, Patricia McFadden, Pennsylvania Institute of Certified Public Accountants, June 18, 2009.

instruction, authoring published articles or books, writing licensing exam items, actively participating in professional or technical societies, or completing patents. Some states hold the authority to approve courses offering professional development hours, whereas others do not. The number of professional development hours awarded varies by activity. Engineers are required to record their professional development hours using standard forms submitted to licensing bodies, and the NCEES encourages random audits of CE completion to ensure that reported CE activities are verifiable (NCEES, 2008). Those failing to meet requirements could face revocation of license, suspension, limitations on licensure, fines, and/or continuing education. Continuing professional competency activities are most often paid for or reimbursed by employers.

CONTINUING EDUCATION FOR PILOTS

The federal pilot certificate does not expire, but to maintain certain flying privileges, pilots are required to abide by specific regulations set forth by the Federal Aviation Administration (FAA). Much like other professions that require CE or continuing professional development (CPD), the FAA requires pilots to have "recent flight experience" before carrying passengers or acting as the pilot in command of an aircraft requiring more than one pilot. For example, a pilot must have made at least three takeoffs and three landings within the preceding 90 days if the intended flight is with passengers or the pilot is in command. If the intended flight is occurring at night, these takeoffs and landings must have been made at night.[3] To maintain instrument flying privileges, a pilot must, among other things, have accomplished six instrument approaches within the 6 months before making an instrument flight. Otherwise, the pilot must undergo an instrument proficiency check with a flight instructor.

Even to fly solo, pilots must undergo a flight review every 2 years, which consists of an hour of flight training and an hour of ground training with a flight instructor. The flight portion consists of maneuvers and procedures that, at the discretion of the flight instructor, demonstrate the pilot can safely exercise the privileges of the pilot certificate. The ground portion consists of reviewing current general operating and flight rules.

It is the pilot's responsibility to document proof of flight experience, such as takeoffs and landings within 90 days, in a pilot log-

---

[3] Electronic Code of Federal Regulations. Title 14 Part 61 § 61.57, June 29, 2009.

book, for example. Flight instructors also make entries in the pilot logbook. The FAA periodically conducts "ramp checks" at airports, where it can ask to see a pilot's certificates and logbook entries.

Companies that employ pilots, such as commercial airlines, may also require pilots to complete training as part of job requirements in addition to FAA-mandated training. Other types of training opportunities exist through traditional classroom training, distance learning, computer-based training, web-based professional networks, and simulations. Simulations are a means to provide pilots with training during adverse conditions and/or to learn new flight techniques while not actually in flight. This training is provided through aviation training companies, such as FlightSafety International, and business aviation associations, such as the International Business Aviation Council. The U.S. military also provides training opportunities. Costs for both mandatory and additional training are incurred by pilots if flying privately or by their employers.

CONTINUING LEGAL EDUCATION

The legal profession has adopted continuing legal education (CLE) as a way to maintain the highest standards for the profession in the midst of constant changes in professional knowledge and to ensure public trust in lawyers. Requirements for CLE are set by individual states and vary from 10 to 15 CLE credits per year, on average (ABA, 2009).

In 2001, the American Bar Association (ABA, 2001) issued the ABA Model Rule for Continuing Legal Education, a guideline document for states to follow as they implement regulatory structures of their own for CLE.[4] The rule describes a structure that would regulate CLE through CLE committees appointed by state supreme courts. CLE committees should include at least one layperson and would be made up entirely of members appointed by state supreme courts (or state bars in states with a unified bar). The CLE requirements apply to all active lawyers; however, the details of individual regulations vary from state to state, and therefore certain approved activities or exceptions to the requirement cannot be considered universal or completely consistent with the ABA Model Rule.[5] Approved activities for CLE include self-study, teaching, writing

---

[4] ABA Model Rule for Continuing Legal Education with Comments, http://www.abanet.org/cle/ammodel.html.

[5] Personal communication, C. Dan Levering, Pennsylvania Continuing Legal Education Board, July 14, 2009.

publications, computer-based educational activities, and in-office law firm CLE. Although states vary in terms of how they assess completion of CLE among lawyers, many require that all active lawyers submit records of their CLE completion every year on a particular date. Although there are generous grace periods for submission, after these extensions expire without proof of CLE completion, state supreme courts may revoke a lawyer's license to practice. The delinquency must then be corrected, and a reinstatement fee of $150 to $500 must be paid.

The ABA Model Rule describes CLE sponsor (analogous to "provider") approval as well. Sponsors apply to their respective CLE committees for accreditation. Approved sponsors may be ABA-accredited law schools or organizations engaged in CLE that, during the 3 years immediately before application, have sponsored six activities that comply with CLE content requirements. The ABA rule stipulates that CLE activities must be of intellectual or practical content and, where possible, include a professional responsibility portion. The activities must contribute directly to lawyers' professional competence, skills, or ethical obligations, and the sponsor must encourage active participation by lawyers as planners, coordinators, authors, panelists, facilitators, or lecturers. CLE sponsors must provide documentation of activities and attendance within 30 days of any request from the CLE committees. Activity leaders must have the necessary practical or academic skills to conduct or facilitate effectively, and a number of other logistical requirements must be met to ensure the adequacy of the facility and method of delivery (e.g., video, audio, web-based) for the CLE activity. CLE employs a unique method of funding: the administrative cost of CLE may be covered by an annual fee established by the CLEC and paid by all active lawyers on the annual reporting date.[6]

PROFESSIONAL DEVELOPMENT FOR TEACHERS

For teachers, "continuous, high-quality professional development is essential to the nation's goal of high standards of learning for every child" (AFT, 2009). High quality professional development will in turn produce high quality teachers,[7] allowing teachers to

---

[6] ABA Model Rule for Continuing Legal Education with Comments.

[7] In order to be a "high quality teacher" under the No Child Left Behind Act, teachers must hold a bachelor's degree, have full state certification, and demonstrate competency in the core academic subjects they teach (U.S. Department of Education, 2006).

assist students in reaching rigorous achievement standards. This section primarily pertains to those teaching kindergarten through twelfth grades in the United States. Most states and the District of Columbia require CE or CPD credits—both terms are used throughout the profession—to maintain certification and licensure (ranging from 90 to 175 hours over 5 years). States are primarily responsible for setting CE or CPD requirements for their teachers. Advanced-level certification is also available to teachers with 3 or more years of teaching experience through the National Board for Professional Teaching Standards (NBPTS). The NBPTS operates an assessment program that awards advanced-level certification in more than 25 areas. The assessment requires teachers to assemble a portfolio of their practices and take a computer-based test of their subject matter knowledge. Pursuing advanced-level certification is a voluntary activity, although some states and districts encourage teachers to earn NBPTS certification and provide salary incentives for teachers who successfully earn the credential (NBPTS, 2009).

School districts ensure that their faculties maintain licensure and certification by reporting data to state education departments, which then report to the U.S. Department of Education, although not all schools are required by law to employ certified teachers (private schools and some chartered schools are exempt). These reporting requirements track the progress of schools and teachers, required under the No Child Left Behind Act of 2001 (NCLB).[8] Under this legislation, all teachers are encouraged to participate in "high quality professional development activities." To finance these activities, state funding has been awarded through grants under NCLB, but in cases where funding has not been granted and prior to the implementation of NCLB, the brunt of the costs were and are faced by the school district (Corcoran, 1995), by states (in the form of subsidies), and by teachers themselves. Providers of CPD include an array of government and nongovernmental organizations, ranging from the U.S. Department of Education to local teacher unions and school districts.

Much like the health professions, teachers are provided with many different options to receive their required CPD units. While professional development opportunities occur through lectures and workshops, e-learning is rapidly growing and can consist of web-based, interactive experiences combining text, audio, and video. The major advantages of e-learning include greater versatility of

---

[8] No Child Left Behind Act of 2001, Public Law 107-110, 107th Congress, 1st Session (January 8, 2002).

the learning materials and methods of dissemination, the potential to build communities from many different geographic regions and sources of expertise, and improvement of teacher retention through direct involvement in their own learning and professional growth. Additionally, teachers may, in some cases, fulfill CE requirements through state-mandated pursuits of further education. For these teachers, their progress through the career ladder is directly linked to ongoing professional development.

LESSONS FOR THE HEALTH PROFESSIONS

Many other professions outside of health care also require their workforces to undergo ongoing training and development to maintain competence and performance, with the overall goal of improving the quality of the workforce. In some professions, CE is mandated at the federal or state levels, whereas it may be voluntary for others. Like the health professions, CE requirements often vary by state and specialty area. CE increasingly includes self-directed learning, e-learning methods, and accomplishments toward professional development; it does not always focus on completion of formal continuing education courses. In some professions, tests of competence, knowledge, and skill are unannounced. Although each profession has tailored CE to its specific needs, lessons can be learned and shared with each other. Various models of learning offer promise for professional behavior and performance and ought to be explored.

REFERENCES

ABA (American Bar Association). 2001. *ABA model rule for continuing legal education.* http://www.abanet.org/cle/ammodel.html (accessed March 25, 2009).
———. 2009. *Summary of MCLE jurisdiction requirements.* http://www.abanet.org/cle/mcleview.html (accessed September 24, 2008).
AFT (American Federation of Teachers). 2009. *Professional development for teachers.* http://www.aft.org/topics/teacher-quality/prodev.htm (accessed June 23, 2009).
AICPA (American Institute of Certified Public Accountants) and NASBA (National Association of State Boards of Accountancy). 2007. *Uniform Accountability Act standards for regulation including substantial equivalency, fifth edition.* New York: AICPA.
Corcoran, T. B. 1995. *Helping teachers teach well: Transforming professional development.* Madison, WI: Consortium for Policy Research in Education.
CSI Construction Education Network. 2008. *State requirements—Engineering.* http://cen.csinet.org/mce_engineering.php (accessed September 23, 2009).
GAO (Government Accountability Office). 2005. *Government auditing standards: Guidance on GAGAS requirements for continuing professional education.* Washington, DC: GAO.

Mele, D. 2005. Ethical education in accounting: Integrating rules, values and virtues. *Journal of Business Ethics* 57:97-109.

NASBA (National Association of State Boards of Accountancy). 2009. *NASBA tools.* http://www.nasbatools.com/display_page?id=6 (accessed June 24, 2009).

NBPTS (National Board for Professional Teaching Standards). 2009. *About us.* http://www.nbpts.org/about_us (accessed June 24, 2009).

NCEES (National Council of Examiners for Engineering and Surveying). 2008. *Continuing professional competency guidelines.* Clemson, SC: NCEES.

U.S. Department of Education. 2006. *The secretary's fifth annual report on teacher quality: A highly qualified teacher in every classroom.* Washington, DC: Office of Postsecondary Education.

VanZante, N. R., and R. B. Fritzsch. 2006. Comparing state board of accountancy CPE requirement with an emphasis on professional ethics requirements. *CPA Journal* 76(10):58.

Appendix E

Workshop Agenda

**Committee on Planning a Continuing Health Care
Professional Education Institute
December 11, 2008**

National Academy of Sciences Building
2100 C Street, N.W., Room 250, Washington, DC

11:15 AM	**Welcome and Introductory Remarks** *Gail Warden, Henry Ford Health System*
11:25 AM	**Understanding the Committee's Charge:** **A Discussion with the Sponsor** *George Thibault, Josiah Macy, Jr. Foundation*
11:45 AM- **12:00 PM**	**Q&A**
12:00-12:45 PM	**Working Lunch** Continue sponsor discussion
12:45-1:00 PM	**Concurrent Activities to Inform the Committee** *Dave Davis, Association of American Medical Colleges* Introduce workshop to (1) review formal continuing education (CE), (2) review a range of alternative interventions, (3) summarize the interprofessional education literature, and (4) review current knowledge in lifelong learning.

1:00-1:15 PM   *Eric Campbell, Institute for Health Policy, Harvard Medical School*
Introduce plan to (1) review what types of continuing medical education (CME) work best, (2) understand the amount of CME that physicians need, (3) review current CME organizational structures, and (4) explore and model alternative CME payment methods.

1:30-1:55 PM   **Q&A**

1:55 PM   **Accreditation, Credentialing and Continuing Education**
1. How can accreditation or credentialing be changed to improve CE?
2. How can CE be strengthened to support professionals' performance?
3. What concerns regarding CE and the Institute of Medicine's (IOM's) study should be brought to the attention of the committee?
Murray Kopelow, Accreditation Council for Continuing Medical Education
Jeanne Floyd, American Nurses Credentialing Center
Peter Vlasses, Accreditation Council for Pharmacy Education
Dwight Hymans, Association of Social Work Boards
David Gibson, Association of Schools of Allied Health Professions
Lisa Robin, Federation of State Medical Boards

3:10-3:40 PM   **Q&A**

3:40 PM   **Perspectives on Continuing Education from Providers and Funders**
1. How does your organization provide for CE activities?
2. How can CE funding and provision be improved from your perspective?
3. Do you believe a continuing education institute is necessary? For what specific roles?
4. How would a continuing education institute change your CE funding or provision roles?

5. What concerns regarding CE and the IOM's study should be brought to the attention of the committee?

Linda Coogle, North American Association of Medical Education and Communication Companies
Cathryn Clary, Pfizer, Inc.

4:00-4:15 PM   **Q&A**

4:15 PM   **Perspectives from Users of Continuing Education**
1. What is the current importance of CE to your daily work?
2. How could CE be changed to make it more useful to you and a more integral part of your practice?
3. What concerns regarding CE and the IOM's study should be brought to the attention of the committee?

Medicine—Michael Moore, Danville Regional Medical Center
Nursing—Patricia Lane, National Black Nurses Association and Inova Fairfax Hospital
Pharmacy—Rebecca Snead, National Alliance of State Pharmacy Associations

4:40-5:00 PM   **Q&A**

5:00 PM   **Continuing Education for Improved Patient Outcomes**
1. What is the current importance of CE for patient well-being?
2. How could CE be improved to benefit patients?
3. What concerns regarding CE and the IOM's study should be brought to the attention of the committee?

John T. James, Patient Safety Advocate
David Swankin, Citizen Advocacy Center

5:15-5:30 PM   **Q&A**

5:30 PM   **ADJOURN**

Appendix F

Committee Member and Staff Biographies

COMMITTEE BIOGRAPHIES

Gail L. Warden, M.H.A., FACHE (*Chair*), serves as president emeritus of Detroit-based Henry Ford Health System and served as its president and chief executive officer (CEO) from 1988 to 2003. He is professor of health management and policy at the University of Michigan, School of Public Health. He is an elected member of the Institute of Medicine (IOM) of the National Academy of Sciences. He served on its Board of Health Care Services, Committee on Quality Health Care in America; chaired the Committee on the Future of Emergency Medicine in the United States; and served two terms on its Governing Council. He is chairman emeritus of the National Quality Forum, chairman emeritus of the National Committee for Quality Assurance, a past chairman of the American Hospital Association, and the chair emeritus of National Center for Healthcare Leadership. He is an emeritus member of the Robert Wood Johnson Foundation Board of Trustees and serves on the RAND Health Board of Advisors. Mr. Warden holds the position of vice chairman and trustee for the Rosalind Franklin University of Medicine and Science's Board of Directors, and he chairs the Detroit Wayne County Health Authority and the Detroit Zoological Society. He is also a director for the National Research Corporation's Board of Directors in Lincoln, Nebraska, and the Picker Institute. He served as a director of Comerica, Inc. from 1990 to 2006. A graduate of Dartmouth College, Mr. Warden holds a master's degree in hospital administration from the University of Michigan. Mr. Warden received an honorary doctorate in public administration from Central Michigan University and an honorary doctorate of humane health care from Rosalind Franklin University of Medicine and Science.

Jako S. Burgers, M.D., Ph.D., is general practitioner, senior consultant at the Dutch Institute for Healthcare Improvement (CBO), and senior researcher at IQ healthcare, Radboud University Nijmegen Medical Centre. Since 1995 he has worked part-time in a general practice in Gorinchem. In the academic year 2008-2009, he was Harkness fellow of the International Program in Health Policy & Practice of the Commonwealth Fund, hosted at the Harvard School of Public Health in Boston. From 1992 to 2002 he worked as a staff member at the Dutch College of General Practitioners and was involved in evidence-based guideline development and continuing medical education programs. From 1998 to 2003 he was coinvestigator in the international AGREE (Appraisal Guidelines Research and Evaluation) project. His thesis "Quality of Clinical Practice Guidelines" was rewarded with the CaRE Award 2002 of the Netherlands School of Primary Care Research. He is trustee of the AGREE Research Trust and founding member of the Guidelines International Network (G-I-N). In 2007-2008, he served as chair of the network and gave several lectures and training workshops on guideline development, adaptation, and implementation in Taiwan, Australia, Saudi Arabia, and Europe.

Linda Burnes Bolton, Dr.P.H., R.N., FAAN, vice president and chief nursing officer at Cedars-Sinai, is the recipient of the American Organization of Nurse Executives (AONE) 2007 Lifetime Achievement Award. As founder of the recently renamed Geri and Richard Brawerman Nursing Institute at Cedars-Sinai, Burnes Bolton oversees development of educational programs in collaboration with nursing schools to increase the supply of nurses, supports research and innovation to improve clinical outcomes, and creates outreach programs to inform students about careers in nursing. Her primary research focuses on women's health, health policy, and organizational development. She has also taken an active leadership role in groundbreaking nursing initiatives such as Transforming Care at the Bedside (TCAB), a national program to improve patient care created and sponsored by the Institute for Healthcare Improvement and the Robert Wood Johnson Foundation. She serves as chair of the National Advisory Committee.

Catherine DeAngelis, M.D., M.P.H., is editor-in-chief of *JAMA, the Journal of the American Medical Association;* senior vice president, Scientific Publications and Multimedia Applications; and professor of pediatrics, Johns Hopkins University, School of Medicine. She received her M.D. from the University of Pittsburgh's School of Medicine, her M.P.H. from the Harvard Graduate School of Public Health (health services administration), and her pediatric specialty training at the Johns Hopkins Hospital. Dr. DeAngelis oversees *JAMA* as well as nine Archives publications and *JAMA*-related website content. Before her appointment with *JAMA*, she was vice dean for academic affairs and faculty, Johns Hopkins University School of Medicine, and from 1994 to 2000, she was editor of *Archives of Pediatrics and Adolescent Medicine*. She also has been a member of the editorial boards of numerous journal. She has authored or edited 11 books on pediatrics and medical education and has published more than 200 original articles, chapters, editorials, and abstracts. Most of her recent publications have focused on conflicts of interest in medicine, on women in medicine, and on medical education. Dr. DeAngelis is a former council member of the National Academy of Sciences, Institute of Medicine; is a fellow of the American Association for the Advancement of Science; and has served as an officer of numerous national academic societies, including past chairman of the American Board of Pediatrics and chair of the Pediatric Accreditation Council for Residency Review Committee of the American Council on Graduate Medical Education. She currently serves on the Advisory Committee to the Director of the National Institutes of Health (NIH) and the Advisory Board of the U.S. Government Accountability Office-Comptroller General.

Robert D. Fox, Ed.D., is professor emeritus of adult and higher education, Department of Educational Leadership, University of Oklahoma, and director of educational research and development, AO Foundation, Davos, Switzerland (part time). His educational background includes doctor of education in adult education, North Carolina State University, 1979; and master of science in adult education, University of Tennessee in Knoxville, 1975. His professional experience includes administrative positions in continuing education at the University of Tennessee and the University of North Carolina Greensboro, director of the Center for Geriatrics and Gerontology at the medical college of East Tennessee State University, and director of the Research Center in Continuing Professional and Higher Education at the University of Oklahoma. His academic positions as full-time faculty have included assistant and associate professor of medical education at the Medical College at East Tennessee State University and professor of adult and higher education at the University of Oklahoma. His research and publications have focused on the process of change in practice and how and why physicians learn. He retired from full-time teaching at the University of Oklahoma in 2008.

Sherry A. Glied, Ph.D., is professor and chair in the Department of Health Policy and Management of Columbia University's Mailman School of Public Health. She holds a Ph.D. in economics from Harvard University. In 1992-1993, she served as a senior economist for health care and labor market policy to the President's Council of Economic Advisers, under President Bush and President Clinton. Her research on health policy has focused on the financing of health care services in the United States. Her book on health care reform, *Chronic Condition,* was published by Harvard University Press in January 1998. She is coauthor (with Richard Frank) of *Better but Not Well: Mental Health Policy in the US Since 1950,* published by Johns Hopkins University Press in July 2006.

Kendall Ho, M.D., FRCPC, is a practicing emergency physician at the Vancouver General Hospital Department of Emergency Medicine. He is the eHealth strategy director, University of British Columbia Faculty of Medicine, and was the immediate past associate dean and director of the Division of Continuing Medical Education of the same university. Dr. Kendall Ho's academic and research interest lies in the domain of technology-enabled knowledge translation (TEKT)—the use of modern information and communication technologies to accelerate the incorporation of evidence into routine practice. His specific research areas in TEKT include the incorporation of adult learning principles into the development of effective and relevant medical education for health professionals; the integration of telecommunication and medical informatics technologies to assist rural and urban health professionals to obtain their continuing education and clinical support on demand; interprofessional team-based practice facilitated by eHealth; and the engagement of the general public using information technologies to promote improved self-management. These areas of interest have led to the development of innovative hands-on workshops to teach physicians skills in using the Internet and personal digital assistants (e.g., Palm Pilots) for professional use, videoconferencing and Internet-based continuing medical educational courses for distributive learning, telemedicine pilot and implementation projects between urban and rural communities, Web 2.0 for health professionals and consumers, and scientific abstracts, editorials, and journal articles on the subjects of medical education, biomedical and health informatics, and telehealth.

Edward F. Lawlor, Ph.D., researches and writes on access to health care, health care reform, policy analysis, and aging. A national Medicare expert, he is the author of *Redesigning the Medicare Contract: Politics, Markets, and Agency.* Dean Lawlor is the founding director of Washington University's Institute for Public Health. He teaches classes on health care policy and services. Prior to joining the Brown School he served as dean at the School of Social Service Administration at the University of Chicago from 1998 to 2004. From 1990 to 1998, he was the director of both the Center for Health Administration Studies and the Graduate Program in Health Administration and Policy at the University of Chicago. He is founding editor of the *Public Policy and Aging Report.* For 10 years Dr. Lawlor was a member and secretary of the Chicago Board of Health, and he has served on numerous policy and advisory bodies in the fields of health care and aging.

David C. Leach, M.D., is the retired CEO of the Accreditation Council for Graduate Medical Education. He was born in Elmira, New York, received a B.A. from the University of Toronto in 1965 and an M.D. from the University of Rochester School of Medicine and Dentistry in 1969. He completed residency training in internal medicine and endocrinology at the Henry Ford Health System in Detroit and is certified in those disciplines. He also had additional training in pediatric endocrinology. He was awarded the Good Samaritan Award by Governor John Engler for his work over 25 years at a Free Clinic in Detroit. He was assistant dean at the University of Michigan for several years, primarily directing the Henry Ford experiences for Michigan students. He was a residency program director and designated institutional official at Henry Ford. He is interested in how physicians acquire competence and are enabled to be authentic practitioners of the art, science, and craft of medicine. He received grant support for innovative curricula for both medical students and residents from the Robert Wood Johnson Foundation and the Pew Charitable Trust. He is interested in chaordic organizations, the teaching of improvement skills, aligning accreditation with emerging health care practices, and the use of educational outcome measures as an accreditation tool. He has received honorary degrees from four medical schools. He is interested in honoring program directors through the Parker J. Palmer Courage to Teach Award. He is a member of the Gold Humanism Honorary Society and is deeply interested in the use of values as well as rules in guiding the behavior of physicians and teachers. He believes that we teach who we are as well as what we are. He is the 2007 recipient of the Abraham Flexner Award for Distinguished Service to Medical Education.

Lucinda Maine, Ph.D., is executive vice president and CEO of the American Association of Colleges of Pharmacy (AACP) in Alexandria, Virginia. AACP member schools are accredited providers of continuing education, and AACP works with the Accrediting Council for Pharmacy Education on standards and guidelines for its accreditation of continuing professional education (CPE) providers. While serving as associate dean for student and alumni affairs at Samford University in Birmingham, Alabama, she directed a program of continuing professional education for pharmacists and other health professionals. She serves as president-elect of the Federation of Associations of Schools of Health Professions and works closely with colleagues from dentistry, nursing, medicine, public health, and allied health professions through this collaboration. AACP does provide educational programs for members but is not an accredited provider of continuing education. She reports no personal conflicts of interest related to continuing education in the health professions.

Paul E. Mazmanian, Ph.D., is a professor at Virginia Commonwealth University with a joint appointment in the Departments of Family Medicine and of Epidemiology and Community Health. He serves as associate dean, Continuing Professional Development and Evaluation Studies, School of Medicine. For 8 years he was chairman of the Master of Public Health Curriculum Committee, leading the program to its first successful academic accreditation. Dr. Mazmanian's research interests include learning and change in physician performance. From 1993 to 1997, he was a member of the Study Section on Health Services Research Dissemination, Agency for Health Care Policy and Research. In 2000, he served as a consultant to the National Research Council, Institute of Medicine, in its efforts to assess prevention and treatment programs associated with violence in families. From August 2004 through February 2005, he consulted with the National Cancer Institute (NCI), helping with NCI's efforts to expedite the translation of new knowledge into clinical solutions. In 2007, he was an invited participant of the Josiah Macy, Jr. Foundation Conference "Continuing Education in the Health Professions."

Dr. Mazmanian is completing his eighth year as editor of the *Journal of Continuing Education in the Health Professions*.

Michael W. Painter, J.D., M.D., a distinguished physician, attorney, health care policy advocate, and 2003-2004 Robert Wood Johnson (RWJF) health policy fellow, is a senior program officer and a senior member of the RWJF Quality/Equality Team. In 2003-2004, Painter was a Robert Wood Johnson Foundation health policy fellow with the office of Senator William H. Frist, M.D., former majority leader. Dr. Painter describes this role as an extraordinary opportunity to employ both his medical and his legal expertise in helping to formulate health care policy at the national level. Prior to that, he was the chief of medical staff at the Seattle Indian Health Board, a community health center serving urban American Indians and Alaska Natives. Dr. Painter led that clinic's award-winning diabetes team. He has a clinical faculty appointment with the University of Washington, Department of Family Medicine. Dr. Painter served as the co-chair for the 2002-2003 Washington State Department of Health Collaborative on Adult Preventive Services and also served as a medical educator and consultant for the Northwest AIDS Education and Training Center. He is a policy advocate at the national, state, and local levels regarding health care issues affecting urban American Indians and Alaska Natives. He is a member of the Cherokee Nation of Oklahoma and the California Bar Association. Dr. Painter earned a B.A. in economics and mathematics from Vanderbilt University, graduating summa cum laude, and is a member of Phi Beta Kappa. He also earned a J.D. from Stanford Law School and an M.D. from the University of Washington. He received his residency training at the Providence Family Medicine Residency in Seattle and is a board-certified family physician.

Wendy Rheault, P.T., Ph.D., is vice president for academic affairs, dean of the College of Health Professions and professor of physical therapy at Rosalind Franklin University of Medicine and Science in North Chicago, Illinois. Dr. Rheault received a B.S. in physical therapy from Queen's University in Kingston, Ontario, Canada, in 1978. In 1981 she received an M.A. in curriculum and instruction from the University of Chicago. In 1989, she was subsequently awarded a Ph.D. (Department of Education) in measurement, evaluation, and statistical analysis, also from the University of Chicago. Accepting the position of vice president of academic affairs in July 2008 while continuing as dean of the College of Health Professions, Dr. Rheault's vice presidential leadership responsibilities encompass the Division of Student Affairs, Learning Resources, Enrollment Services, Educational Affairs, and the Education and Evaluation Center. In her capacity as vice president, Dr. Rheault is also an ad hoc member of the Academic Committee of the Board.

Marie E. Sinioris, M.P.H., is president and CEO of the National Center for Healthcare Leadership (NCHL), a not-for-profit organization whose mission is to be a catalyst to ensure that high quality, relevant, and accountable health management leadership is available to meet the needs of twenty-first century health care. Ms. Sinioris, a co-founder of NCHL, provides overall strategic direction and leads NCHL's national research and demonstration programs on health leadership competencies and best practices that contribute to leadership and organizational excellence. The adoption of best practices is accelerated through shared learning and benchmarking within NCHL's nationally recognized Leadership Excellence Networks (LENS). NCHL's goal is to improve the health status of the entire country through effective health care management leadership. Prior to assuming this national role, Ms. Sinioris was president and CEO of Arc Ventures, LLC, a diversified health care company affiliated with Rush-Presbyterian-St. Luke's Medical Center in Chicago, Illinois. As president, she directed the development and record growth of Arc's diversified portfolio of businesses. While with Rush, she also served as corporate vice president of strategic planning and senior vice president and chief operating officer of Rush Health Plans, a health maintenance organization-preferred provider organization (HMO-PPO) covering more than a quarter of a million people in the Chicago metropolitan area. She is a professor in the Department of Health Systems Management at Rush University.

STAFF BIOGRAPHIES

Cassandra Cacace is a senior program assistant for the Board on Health Care Services, assisting on a variety of projects, including the Committee on Continuing Education, the Committee on Resident Duty Hours and Patient Safety, and the Forum on the Science of Health Care Quality Improvement and Implementation. She provides administrative and research support to the teams, as well as logistical support for all committee meetings. Prior to the IOM, Cassandra worked as a research associate at Oxford Outcomes, a health care consulting firm, where she performed outcomes research on a variety of health conditions. She is currently pursuing her master's degree in health policy from the George Washington University School of Public Health and Health Services.

Samantha M. Chao, M.P.H., is a program officer at the Institute of Medicine, working on issues related to health care quality. Most recently she directed the Forum on the Science of Health Care Quality Improvement and Implementation, which brought together leaders in the field to discuss methods to improve the quality and value of health care through the strengthening of research. She previously staffed the Pathways to Quality Health Care Series that reviewed performance measures to analyze health care delivery, evaluated Medicare's Quality Improvement Organization Program, and assessed pay for performance and its potential role in Medicare. Prior to joining the IOM, she completed a master's degree in health policy with a concentration in management at the University of Michigan, School of Public Health. As part of her studies, she interned with the American Heart Association and the Michigan Department of Community Health.

Roger C. Herdman, M.D., was born in Boston, Massachusetts, and attended Phillips Exeter Academy, graduating in 1951; he received degrees from Yale University, B.S., magna cum laude, Phi Beta Kappa, in 1955 and Yale University School of Medicine, M.D., in 1958. He interned at the University of Minnesota and was a medical officer in the U.S. Navy from 1959 to 1961. Thereafter, he completed a residency in pediatrics and continued with a medical fellowship in immunology-nephrology at Minnesota. He held positions of assistant professor and professor of pediatrics at the University of Minnesota and the Albany Medical College between 1966 and 1979. In 1969, he was appointed director of the New York State Kidney Disease Institute in Albany. During 1969-1977 he served as deputy commissioner of the New York State Department of Health responsible for research, departmental health care facilities, and the Medicaid program at various times. In 1977, he was named New York State's director of public health. From 1979 until joining the U.S. Congress's Office of Technology Assessment (OTA), he was a vice president of the Memorial Sloan-Kettering Cancer Center in New York City. In 1983, he was named assistant director of OTA and then acting director and director from January 1993 to February 1996. After the closure of OTA, he joined the National Academy of Sciences' Institute of Medicine as a senior scholar and subsequently served as director of the National Cancer Policy Board and the National

Cancer Policy Forum. He is now the director of the Board on Health Care Services.

Bernadette McFadden, M.Sc., joined the Board on Health Care Services as a research associate in November 2008. Prior to joining the IOM, she completed a master's degree in social research at Trinity College, Dublin. As part of her studies, she was employed by Dublin City Council's Homeless Agency, where she edited a volume of essays on homelessness in Ireland and wrote a report on how the city's management of public space impacts homeless persons. Her interests in health policy developed while employed as an Ameri-Corps teacher in the Atlanta Public Schools system. She graduated summa cum laude, Phi Beta Kappa, from Dickinson College in Carlisle, Pennsylvania. While in central Pennsylvania, she interned with the Executive Policy Office of the Pennsylvania Department of Health and served as a board member on the United Way of Cumberland County.

Adam Schickedanz is a senior medical student at the University of California, San Francisco (UCSF); a graduate of Washington University in St. Louis (B.A., 2003); and a Boston native. At UCSF Adam has developed a clinical focus in urban underserved patient care, while also advancing interests in professionalism and cultural competency in medical education, novel approaches to clinician-patient communication in medical decision making (particularly at the end of life), and the intersections of education and health. He interned with the Board on Health Care Services and was a Mirzayan policy fellow through May 2009, when he returned to UCSF to complete his M.D.